the
fast
beach
diet

the fast beach diet

MIMI SPENCER
with a foreword by
Dr Michael Mosley

If you are in reasonable health, short fasts (which will always, don't forget, include the Fast Diet's calorie allowance) should be fine. If you are on medication of any description, please see your doctor first. There are certain groups for whom fasting is not advised. Type 1 diabetics are included in this list, along with anyone suffering from an eating disorder. If you are already extremely lean, do not fast. Children should never fast, so this is a plan for over-18s only. Pregnant women should eat according to government guidelines and not limit their daily calorie intake. Similarly, if you have an underlying medical condition, visit your GP, as you would before embarking on any weight-loss regime.

Published in 2014 by Short Books
3A Exmouth House
Pine Street
EC1R 0JH

10 9 8 7 6 5 4 3 2 1

A CIP catalogue record for this book
is available from the British Library.

ISBN 978-1-78072-224-5

Printed in Great Britain by CPI Group (UK) Ltd.
Croydon, CR0 4YY

contents

foreword

The Fast way to better health

Intermittent Fasting is, without doubt, one of the hottest new approaches to weight loss on the planet. When *The Fast Diet* was published in January 2013, Mimi and I could never have imagined the response it would get. It quickly became an international phenomenon, and has since been embraced by celebrities like Beyoncé and Benedict Cumberbatch ('You have to, for *Sherlock*'). *One Foot in the Grave* star Richard Wilson told a newspaper that he had lost 12lb on the diet in just five weeks. 'The great thing is that the fasting days are tough but you know that the next day you can eat.' Even the new slim-line Chancellor of the Exchequer, George Osborne, is rumoured to be on it.

I am passionate about IF because I find the science compelling and because there is such good evidence of potential health benefits. I am also convinced by the dramatic effects it has had on my own body. By way of background, for those of you who have not read the original book, two years ago I was an overweight middle-aged man, weighing in at around 85kg (13st 3lb), with a 36-inch waist. I was mildly embarrassed about the spare tyre round my gut, but not embarrassed enough to do anything about it.

Then I went to my doctor with a minor complaint and as part of the examination she suggested I have a routine blood test. When the results came back she told me that I was a Type 2 diabetic, with a fasting glucose of around 7.2 mmol/l. This was a nasty shock as my father had passed away at a relatively early age; when he died he was suffering from a range of diseases, including Type 2 diabetes, heart failure, prostate cancer and what I suspect was early dementia.

Rather than start on medication, I began researching alternative approaches and came across Intermittent Fasting. I decided to make a documentary on the subject; in the course of making the film *Eat, Fast, Live Longer*, I tried various different forms of IF, ranging from doing five days of almost total calorie restriction to alternate-day fasting (where you cut your calories every other day). Eventually I settled on a pattern I found easy to stick to, which I called the 5:2 diet.

On a Monday and a Thursday I ate a quarter of my normal calorie intake, going down from around 2400 to 600 calories a day. In 12 weeks on this diet I lost 9kg (nearly 20lb) and 4 inches off my waist. My body fat went down from 28% to 21%. My blood glucose fell to healthy levels. I also began to sleep better (I lost fat around my neck and stopped snoring).

I then began combining the IF with an intermittent exercise regime ('Fast Exercise') and soon began to see the beginnings of a six-pack. I can now fit into a suit I haven't worn for 30 years.

As our website testifies, this is an experience that has been replicated thousands of times over. We now have feedback from countless people who have embarked on the 5:2 Fast Diet and found it to be positively life-changing.

So why has Mimi written a new book? Well, the original book laid out the science behind IF and gave useful tips on how to do it. What it didn't do was produce a structured regime, one that would ensure fat loss over a comparatively short period of time. *The Fast Beach Diet* is an adjunct, if you like, designed to complement the original *Fast Diet* – a short-term, faster solution for those of you who perhaps have a fat-loss deadline to meet.

The original book also made very little reference to exercise. Although studies show that low intensity exercise, like jogging, is unlikely to lead to weight loss (people tend to compensate by eating more), there is plenty of evidence that a combination of calorie restriction and exercise will lead to more sustained weight loss than either done alone. *The Fast Beach Diet* includes useful sections on how to get fitter and better toned in just a few minutes a day.

Best of all, Mimi has produced a range of new and tasty recipes for your Fast Days. I have begun to work my way through them and can testify that they are full of flavour as well as hunger-killing fibre and protein.

I greatly enjoyed reading this book and learned something new from doing so. I hope you do too.

Dr Michael Mosley

chapter 1

The Fast Diet revisited... and an invitation to the beach

'A year from now, you will wish you started today'

There are many good reasons to start the Fast Diet. You may be inspired by your sister or your best friend, your dad or your doctor. You may have decided you want to cut your risk of age-related disease. You may want to reduce your cholesterol, boost your brain, improve your mood, lower your blood pressure, lengthen your life.

Or you may just want to look good in a swimsuit.

I say 'just'. But looking good and (more importantly) feeling good about your body is no mere vanity project. It can have a real emotional impact on a life. I'm reminded of one Fast Dieter who told me that, after years of fruitless yo-yo dieting, six months of 5:2 had given her enough body confidence to go to the local baths and swim with her young daughter for the first time ever. That's not vanity. It's the glorious stuff of life.

Not long ago, a magazine survey found that women think about their bodies every 15 minutes (which is, apparently, more than men think about sex). There are times of the year, of course, when we put ourselves under greater scrutiny still. On the beach, in summer, in our shorts and bikinis, we think about the shape we're in even more often – a constant background hum, the helicopter moaning overhead. Men may not bang on about it quite as much, but they tend to be just as aware as T-shirt weather creeps up to ambush those hibernating pecs and paunches.

So now is the time to act. The beach beckons and this is your call to arms. The most challenging weeks of the year may be looming on the sun-kissed horizon, but that's no reason to bury your head in the sand or collapse into a kaftan for cover. We have a plan. It is called the Fast Beach Diet. Think of it as '5:2, the Next Generation'. It promises to shake things up, with a wealth of new tips, tricks and takes to help you break the plateau, make the leap and reboot your 5:2 for summer. In the words of the late, great Janis Joplin, we're gonna try… just a little bit harder. But first, let's recap on the original Fast Diet – what it is and how it works.

What is the Fast Diet?

It may be radical, but the Fast Diet is also wonderfully eco-nomical with its rules. I like that *The Times* has called it the 'haiku diet' – a pithy, almost poetic agenda. All you really need to know is that:

• You eat normally for five days a week and then, for the other two days, you consume a quarter of your normal calorie intake – around 600 calories for men, 500 for women. So, it is not total 'fasting', but a modified version

• It is not continual fasting, but intermittent. Our experience is that non-consecutive Fast Days work best, though you can do them back to back if you prefer

• Most people divide their calorie allowance between breakfast and an evening meal, aiming for a lengthy 'Fasting Window' between meals. But you can skip breakfast and have a more substantial evening meal containing your whole calorie quota if it better suits your day

• It does matter what you eat on a Fast Day: plan your calorie quota by sticking, as the recipes in chapter 7 do, to the Fast Diet mantra: 'Mostly Plants and Protein'. That way, you'll stay fuller longer and get adequate nutrients in your diet

Why 5:2?

In the beginning, Michael tried several different fasting regimes; the one he settled on as the most realistic and sustainable was five days off, two days on, which meant that the majority of the time was spent free from calorie-counting. On this regime, in 12 weeks Michael lost more than 20lb of body fat and his blood glucose fell to a healthy level. I lost 22lb and returned to my pre-motherhood body weight (and, more importantly, shape).

That was only a little over 18 months ago. We're still learning about the true long-term benefits of Intermittent Fasting, and we don't, as yet, have a comprehensive account of potential pitfalls, particularly why some people flourish on 5:2 and others may find it harder. It may be that there is no 'one size fits all'. What we do know is that thousands of people have followed the Fast Diet, lost weight, gained health and found it surprisingly sustainable, effective and life-affirming. New studies are underway and we hope to bring together the latest thinking in a fully updated new edition to be published in 2015.

So where's the catch?

Really, there isn't one. The Fast Diet, don't forget, is simply a modern take on an ancient idea. Fasting, in one form or another, has been practised for centuries by most of the great religions, and if done properly seems to be extremely safe. There is no evidence of significant side effects (though some people may experience headaches and constipation, particularly at first; these can generally be prevented by drinking lots of water or calorie-free fluids, such as black coffee and herbal tea, and eating foods rich in fibre).

Indeed, the Fast Diet has helped to debunk some of the myths that have developed around the way we eat in the West – for instance that:

• You need to eat whenever you feel hungry

• Eating every few hours will increase your metabolic rate

• If you don't eat every few hours your blood sugar will fall and you will feel faint

None of these widely held beliefs is backed by science. You will discover that short bouts of hunger are manageable and soon pass. Similarly, there is no metabolic advantage to spreading your calories over the day, nor is there any evidence that short periods without food will cause your blood glucose to plunge to seriously low levels. Most nights, don't forget, you happily go 12 hours without eating and many people feel fine with a late breakfast, especially on a Sunday when the start can be in delicious slow-mo.

Should you be sceptical?

Michael and I certainly were. After all, anyone who has ever gone on a conventional diet knows that they are hard work; they may deliver results in the short term, but then life gets in the way – we're soon bored and the weight creeps back on. We've found, however, that the 5:2 Fast Diet does work – for exactly the reason that other diets don't: there is none of the boredom, frustration or serial denial that characterises standard diet plans; eating is still a pleasure; there's no cutting of food groups, no pathologising of eating. And indeed, even the turbo version laid out here is full of forgiveness, generosity of spirit and the crucial adaptability required to fit it into a busy life.

A word on the benefits of Intermittent Fasting

The reason behind IF – briefly but severely restricting the number of calories you consume – is that it 'fools' your body into thinking it is in a potential famine situation and that it needs to switch from go-go mode to maintenance mode. Fasting is the shock that resets the clock. Its many benefits include:

• Fat loss of 1-2lb a week

• A reduction in a hormone called IGF-1, which means that you are reducing your risk of a number of age-related diseases

• The switching-on of repair genes

• Improvements in cardiovascular health and cholesterol levels

• A rest for your pancreas, boosting the effectiveness of the insulin it produces in response to elevated blood glucose

• Metabolic changes that tweak your body into burning fat and increase its insulin sensitivity; this in turn will reduce your risk of obesity, diabetes, heart disease and cognitive decline

• Increased levels of neurotrophic factor in the brain, which should make you more cheerful, even when contemplating your summer swimsuit

The Fast Diet and weight loss

While clinical studies into IF in general, and 5:2 in particular, are still in their early stages, there's a great deal of convincing anecdotal evidence that the approach can be startlingly effective for many people. Anecdote, as Michael often says, makes poor science, but it does tell a story. Many thousands of people have adopted the plan and witnessed significant improvements in their weight, cholesterol and general health, and have gone on to post their success stories online (we have included just a fraction of these in the testimonials chapter at the back of this book). We regularly meet people in the street and see friends and family who've lost weight and gained health. My father, for instance, has lost four stone over the course of a year on the Fast Diet. That's about the weight of an eight-year-old child. I can now get my arms all the way around him when we hug hello. It's a seismic change, and a joy to behold.

HOW FASTING TARGETS FAT

What people sometimes forget in their drive to 'lose weight' is what they really want to lose is not weight as such, but fat. Carrying excess fat is not just a bummer on the beach; it's bad for your health.

Here's what we know about the effect IF has on fat:
• It achieves a gradual weight loss – and it's almost all fat
• It increases fat burn. More of the calories you use for fuel during a fast come from fat stores than muscle. A study from Nottingham University[1] found that the proportion of energy obtained from fat rose progressively over 12-72 hours of fasting, until almost all the energy being used was coming from stored fat
• When we eat, we use the carbohydrate and fat supplied by the food for fuel, instead of tapping into our stored fat reserves. Constant grazing may be what's keeping fat from being burned – and fasting is one way to release it
• Interestingly, the heavier you are, the more likely it is that fasting will lead to substantial fat loss with muscle being spared
• A bonus for Intermittent Fasters is that it seems to lead not just to fat loss generally, but specifically to fat loss around the gut – this is the visceral fat and is particularly dangerous because it increases your risk of heart disease and diabetes
• One reason why it's important to preserve as much muscle mass as possible is that muscle is metabolically active. Lean tissue burns calories, even at rest

So why the Fast Beach Diet?

The Fast Diet's USP seems to be its high level of compliance: we do it and we stick with it because most of the time, we're not thinking about dieting at all. But some fasters want to boost the process at certain times of year. You may be one of those for whom the 5:2 has not proved the magic bullet you hoped for. Others among you may want to nudge yourself off a plateau and budge any reluctant pounds that are hanging on in there despite your adherence to 5:2.

I've written this book to be used as a primer for the summer holidays; the idea is to start the six-week regime in May, June or July, in good time for take-off (that's clothes, not planes). The longer, brighter days and fresher produce of late spring and early summer make it an ideal time to embark or improve upon a weight-loss programme. And, as we've already established, there's nothing like an approaching bikini – or T-shirt – to make you think twice about that piece of pie.

That said, the principles of the turbo-driven 5:2 diet laid out here are applicable at almost any time of the year. You might like to use its additional hints and ideas if you are preparing to get married, if you have a big event coming up, if you're starting a new phase in your life, if you're ready to lose some baby weight, or if you've had a particularly sedentary and stodgy couple of months (after Christmas perhaps).

You may, of course, be coming to *The Fast Beach Diet* cold, without having read or acted upon the original book.

This book is an adjunct. Think of it as a boot camp for the 5:2. It is a condensed, modified programme of greater intensity with the aim of helping you achieve a reasonable target weight in a six-week period. Note now that on the Fast Beach Diet, you will be encouraged to step it up – to get a tad tougher, a bit bolder, with your Fast Diet. But this extra commitment is intended to be short-lived. Just a bit more effort. For just six weeks.

Why six weeks?

In truth, the six-week figure is fairly arbitrary. I have used my own experience and a 25-year career in the fashion and body-shape business, together with what I have learned from many other dieters, to come up with a reasonable period during which I believe the average individual – someone with a little willpower and plenty of good intentions – can commit to and concentrate on a more intense 5:2 regime. It hinges on attention span and compliance; six weeks should be enough time to see measurable results without boredom setting in. It's also, by happy coincidence, about the length of time we usually give ourselves to prepare mentally and physically for our summer holidays… the Six Week Sprint to the pool.

You may choose to extend the Fast Beach Diet, perhaps to two months. But be clear: it is only meant to be a short-term option; afterwards, you should return to the classic Fast Diet rules, without undue concern for calories on a non-Fast Day. Remember: it is this flexible and sociable foundation that lends the Fast Diet its psychological advantage.

If the Fast Beach Diet seems unnecessarily faddish to you, or if you're not keen on a 'fast-fix' message, if you treasure the absolute simplicity of the original Fast Diet – well, I empathise and understand. Just stick with your original 5:2 Fast Diet. This book is aimed at people who want a short-term booster plan to get them from A (the sofa) to B (the beach) by undertaking a reasonable but more vigorous protocol. It's not designed to be a 'forever plan' like the 5:2. It's the Fast Diet, just a bit faster. So are you in? Here's what to expect…

The Fast Beach Diet includes:

• A clear six-week plan to encourage fat loss

• Plateau-busting techniques to jump-start the 5:2 and make it work for you

• Mindfulness methods to help you tough out a fast and eat with understanding every day

• Habit-changing ideas to sharpen up on non-Fast Days

• A High Intensity Training (HIT) exercise programme for fitness and fat loss, achievable in just a few minutes a day

• Lots of brand-new, calorie-counted summer recipes, with plenty of healthy, speedy ideas for busy days

• Motivation, meal plans and 5:2 support to rev up your Fast Diet and help get you beach-fit for summer

When should you start?

If you do not have an underlying medical condition, and if you are not an individual for whom fasting is proscribed (see page 4), then there really is no time like the present. But first, a bit of prep.

chapter 2

Getting started

Know yourself

Weigh in and plot your progress

Before the off, you really need to understand what shape you're in. It's time for a reality check; shrug off the winter layers and see what lies beneath. While noting the aphorism that 'good health is not about weight; weight is an indicator of good health', it is worth knowing your current weight, monitoring your progress, and having a target in mind.

• Ideally use a scale that measures body-fat percentage as well as weight, since what you really want to see is body-fat levels fall. Women tend to have more body fat than men. A man with body fat of more than 25% is considered overweight. For a woman, it's 30%

• Though not without controversy, the easiest way to gauge which weight category you fall into (healthy; overweight; obese) is by calculating your Body Mass Index (BMI). This is your weight (in kgs) divided by your height (in metres) squared. Do note that a BMI score takes no account of body type, age or ethnicity, so should be treated with informed caution. Still, if you need a number, this is the one to watch

• Use the BMI equation to calculate an upper and lower limit for your desirable target weight. So, for example, I am 5'7" (1.70m). A normal, healthy BMI is between 18.5 and 24.9, so a reasonable weight for my height would be somewhere between 53.5kg (about 8st 4lb) and 72kg (about 11st 3lb). This is obviously a fairly wide range: it's up to you to decide what's right and what's possible

• If you are significantly heavier than your target weight, see your doctor before embarking on the Fast Beach Diet. It's important that any weight-loss or exercise programme is safe, and heavier individuals should seek medical advice before starting

• Measure your waist as an indicator of internal 'visceral' fat: male or female, ideally your waist should be less than half your height. Most people underestimate their waist size by about two inches because they rely on trouser size. Instead, measure your waist by putting the tape measure around your belly button

• You may choose to have your bloods tested for fasting glucose (an important measure of fitness and predictor of future health), cholesterol and triglycerides. Your doctor should be able to do this

Be realistic

Precipitous weight loss is not advised, so be sensible and

choose a target that seems reasonable. Make a plan. Write it down, recognising that dieters who keep an honest account of what they eat and drink are more likely to lose the pounds and keep them off. Try using the pull-out chart included in this book. I suggest weighing yourself twice a week, first thing in the morning, preferably the day after a fast. You might like to use a tracker – the Fast Beach Diet app will do this, or try the tracker at www.thefastdiet.co.uk to plot your progress.

Remember, everyone is different. There will almost certainly be fluctuations in your weight. Some weeks, you may achieve impressive weight loss. Others, you may grind to a halt. If you have not been on the Fast Diet already, you may find that in the early weeks of the Fast Beach Diet your weight drops quite quickly (some of this will be water). What you're looking for is a downward trajectory, with an average weight loss of about 2lb a week; but don't get hung up on the day-to-day numbers. Realise that the goal here is HEALTH. Looking good in a swimsuit is nice. But a long and healthy life is so much better.

Prepare yourself

As 5:2 devotees well know, it's worth spending a little time getting ready for a Fast Day. Don't over-think it, but it does matter that you have at least considered what, how and when you're likely to eat – not least because we live in an 'obesogenic environment' with opportunities to consume calories at every turn. If you are embarking on the six-week Fast Beach Diet, here's how to maximise your chances of success...

Plan your Fast Days

• Eliminate illicit food stashes: empty your snack drawer at work; clear the house of junk food. Those biscuits may look innocuous, but they're out to trip you up

• Shop on non-Fast Days, so as not to taunt yourself with undue temptation

• Stock up on herbal teas and healthy low-cal drinks (see pages 60-61)

• Remember: if you don't buy it, you can't forage for it, so shop wisely. Buy more fresh vegetables and have them handy

• Have a clear idea of your favourite Fast Day foods, remembering to embrace Variety and Volume – the double V key to staying fuller longer

• Make good Fast Day food in advance and have it ready in the freezer. Keep it simple, aiming for flavour without effort (for great recipe ideas, see pages 103-41)

• Don't bump into food by accident – if you're in a rush, you'll never make yourself an interesting salad. You'll stop off at the petrol station and buy a packet of M&Ms

• Be flexible – work out your plan according to your needs, the shape of your day, your family, your commitments, your preferences. You may like to eat once, or twice, first thing or last. Some individuals prefer to be told exactly what to eat and when; others like a more informal approach. That's fine. It's enough to simply stick to the basic method – 500 or 600 calories a day, with as long a 'window without food' as possible, twice a week – and you'll gain the plan's multiple benefits

Clear the diary

Begin on a day when you feel strong, purposeful, calm and committed. Tell friends and family that you're starting the Fast Beach Diet: as we'll see, once you make a public commitment, you are much more likely to stick with it. Avoid high days, holidays and days when you know food will be the focus. But do keep busy; it's the best way to zip through a Fast Day and on to tomorrow without dwelling too much on the process. Some women may find fasting more challenging on the days preceding a period; we don't yet have any clear human studies on the impact of IF on the menstrual cycle, but if you feel this may be the case for you, perhaps fast on the days following the start of your period, not before.

Clear your mind

Not as dippy as it sounds: the success of your Fast Beach Diet will depend largely on getting your mind in gear at the outset. Think positive. Stay strong. Be bold. Have a clear idea of what you want, why you want it and what the hurdles may be. To help yourself, answer the following questions before the off:

• What's my motivation?

- What's my weakness?

- What's my goal?

Write down the answers and put them somewhere handy – tucked in your purse, stuffed in the bread bin, stuck inside the front door with Blu-Tack… Once you're off the blocks, you may well find, as many Fast Dieters do, that occasional fasting makes you feel more connected, happier in yourself. There's plenty more on motivation and mindfulness in the pages ahead.

chapter 3

Your Fast Days in practice

So. Today's the day. Six weeks until the great reveal. We all do it, don't we? We calculate a reasonable interval between now and the first beach outing, a window of opportunity and diligence that, in theory, should get us swimsuit-ready in a great six-week leap. Women apparently plan to lose an average of 8lb in the run-up to a holiday. The operative word here is 'plan'. I suspect that the reason everyone looks so despondent in the departure lounge at Gatwick is that they've all been bitterly disappointed by the scales that very morning. But with the Fast Beach Diet, you're stacking the odds in your favour. Stay focused. Stay firm. This, you can do.

Which days to choose?

It really doesn't matter. It's your life, and you'll know which days will suit you best. Monday is an obvious choice for many, perhaps because it is more manageable, psychologically and practically, to gear yourself up at the beginning of a new week, particularly if it follows a sociable weekend. For that reason, fasters might choose to avoid Saturdays and Sundays, when family lunches and brunches, dinner dates and parties make calorie-cutting a bore. Thursday would then make a sensible second Fast Day, chiming, if such things appeal, with the teachings of the Prophet Mohammed, who is understood to have fasted the second and fifth days of the week. But be flexible; don't force yourself to fast when it feels wrong. If you're particularly stressed, off-colour, tired or peevish on a day that you have designated a fast, try again another day. Adapt. Do, however, aim for a pattern. That way, over the six-week period, your fasts will become familiar, a low-key habit you accept and embrace.

When to eat?

Go with a timetable that suits you. Some fasters appreciate the convenience and simplicity of a single 500/600-calorie evening meal, allowing them to ignore food entirely for most of the day; some people say they actually feel hungrier during the day if they have breakfast. Having just one meal, as late in the day as possible, will clearly intensify the fast – allowing your body a longer period in which to be in a fasted state. Others prefer to eat breakfast and then avoid food for a Fasting Window of around 12 hours until supper.

Since it is the fasted state that is so beneficial to us, eating lots of small meals is likely to significantly reduce the benefits, particularly if you graze on carbohydrates. Mark Mattson at the National Institute on Aging agrees that eating the 500/600 calories at one meal is better than eating several smaller meals over the course of the day. It is, however, only 'better' if you actually do it. Compliance is critical, so experiment a bit and opt for a pattern that works for you. Remember that over time, as you get used to the diet, your body should acclimatise to periods of fasting; so keep your personal pattern flexible and adjust to a more lengthy Fasting Window when you feel able. Stay alert and tweak the regime to suit your needs.

What to eat

Aim to have food that makes you feel satisfied, but stays firmly within the 500/600-calorie allowance – the best options to achieve this are foods that contain lean protein, and foods with a low Glycaemic Index – for more on this, see page 46. So, stick to the Fast Day mantra: 'Mostly Plants and Protein'.

The Fast Diet does not recommend boycotting carbs entirely, nor does it suggest living permanently on a high-protein diet. We certainly don't advise eating protein to the exclusion of all else on a Fast Day, but you do require an adequate quantity, for muscle health, cell maintenance, endocrinal regulation and immunity. Protein is satiating too, so it's a valuable part of your calorie quota. We recommend that you boost the protein content of your diet on Fast Days, so that it makes up a greater proportion of your diet on just those days. The best advice is to stick to recommended governmental guidelines, which allow for a (quite generous) 50g per day. Go for 'good protein' – steamed white fish, eggs, prawns, tofu and plant protein from nuts, seeds and pulses (which are also full of fibre and act as bulking agents on a hungry day). When it comes to veg, bring in the Double Vs – plenty of Volume, plenty of Variety.

What does fasting feel like?

If it has been a while since you have experienced hunger, you'll probably find that eating no more than 500 or 600 calories in a day is a mild challenge, at least initially. Intermittent Fasters do report that the process becomes significantly easier with time, particularly as they witness results in the mirror and on the scales. Have faith: your mission is to get through the day.

Getting past the lows... and feeling the highs

There is no reason to be alarmed by benign, occasional, short-term hunger. Given base-level good health, it will do you no harm at all. Your body is designed to go without food for longish periods, even if it has lost the skill through years of routine picking and snacking.

Remember that the diet you may have been used to – a typical Western grazing diet – is almost designed to make you feel hungry, so much so that hunger becomes the white noise of daily life. Try to recognise that what you feel as 'hunger' can be a learned reaction to external cues – it's often, as we'll see in chapter 4, 'emotional hunger', rather than a true physiological state. There are ways to circumvent the feeling: the real trick is to eat food which keeps you feeling fuller longer. This means some protein. This means slow-burn, low-GI fuel. This means bulk from plants.

In any case, you're unlikely to be troubled by hunger at all until well into a Fast Day. Fasters also report that the feeling of perceived hunger comes in waves; it will pass. You have absolute power to conquer feelings of hunger, simply by steering your mind, riding those waves, choosing to do something else; perhaps drink a herbal tea, go for a walk, get stuck into a sudoku or a movie or a particularly gripping novel. This is an acquired skill, and you'll discover plenty of ways to obtain it in the chapters to come. Some people (Matthew McConaughey among them, apparently) swear that brushing their teeth stops them feeling peckish... Do whatever works for you.

After a few weeks' practising IF, people generally report that their sense of hunger is diminished. So, take heart. On a Fast Day, refrain, restrain, divert and distract yourself. Before you know it, you've retrained your brain and hunger's off the menu.

One of the reasons that the Fast Diet has proved so sustainable for so many is the simple realisation that 'tomorrow's another day'. There's boundless psychological comfort in the fact that your fasting will only ever be a brief break from food. On the Fast Beach Diet, you will still be eating 'normally' on non-Fast Days: you'll simply be eating with more awareness than you might on the traditional Fast Diet, using techniques to ensure that your food choices are absolutely the best you can make.

Bear in mind, too, that fasters regularly report that the

food with which they 'break their fast' tastes great; my mother-in-law calls this 'hunger sauce' – and if you've never tasted it, you're in for a treat. There's nothing like a bit of delayed gratification to make good things taste even better.

Fast Day tips

Stay hydrated

Drink plenty of water. Get into the habit of drinking a glass of water before and after Fast Day meals. And drink water when you feel hungry too (it really does help; the stomach is a simple beast); it will also stop you mistaking thirst for hunger. At the most basic level, drinking water keeps your mouth occupied when it would otherwise be anticipating a snack. Supplement your water intake with herbal tea, black coffee, miso soup – but not juice which, as we'll see on page 57, can rack up the sugars. For more great summertime Fast Beach Diet drinks, see pages 60-61.

Axe the snacks

Remember, your aim is to secure a food-free breathing space for your body. All calories count on a Fast Day, and your objective is to achieve as long a Fasting Window as possible. Having a complete moratorium on snacking actually makes the process easier to handle: if 'no means no', then you avoid questions or calorie calculations. No nibbles, no quibbles. But if you absolutely must snack, make it a good one: have berries, an apple, a carrot. See page 137 for a list of Fast-friendly calorie-counted snacks.

Keep your perspective

Going to 510 calories (or 615 for a man) won't hurt – it won't obliterate a fast. But while there's no particular 'magic' to 500 or 600 calories, do try to stick broadly to these numbers; you need clear parameters to make the strategy effective in the medium term. And stay positive. Don't be disheartened if you plateau and don't lose weight in any given week; weight loss is your bonus, not your sole objective.

chapter 4

Introducing the
Fast Diet Max

As we established in the original *Fast Diet* book, in order to be effective, any weight-loss regime must be sustainable over the long haul. 'To work at all,' I wrote back then, 'any weight-loss strategy has to be tolerable, organic and innate, not some spurious add-on that makes you feel awkward and self-conscious, the dietary equivalent of uncomfortable shoes...' We know that one of the keys to the success of the 5:2 Fast Diet is compliance – we do it gladly because the commitment is only occasional and always leavened by the prospect of a day of normal eating tomorrow.

The Fast Beach Diet takes a slightly different tack. Think of it as a jump-start. A reboot. It's the turbo-drive button that takes you off cruise control. The idea is to commit to a six-week modified programme, knowing that you can soon return to the familiar territory of the classic 5:2. You may want to use it in the run-up to a holiday, a wedding, a moment when you want to shine, a day that demands that you look your slimline best. It's for people who may feel they have got a bit stuck; just as having a dry January or growing a moustache for November has become part of many people's annual calendar, so the Fast Beach Diet can be your short-term, souped-up strategy for summer. Its approach is three-pronged, based on ways to:

• Tighten up on Fast Days

• Toughen up on non-Fast Days, and

• Tune in on any day

You may choose to include most of the suggestions here, or just a handful of them. If you want a shorthand checklist of all the Fast Beach Diet hints, tips and techniques, you'll find one at the end of the six-week diet planner included in this book. First, it's time to rev up your Fast Days.

Tighten up on Fast Days

The simple premise of the Fast Diet requires you to cut back hard on calories for two days a week, and it's entirely possible that this is more than enough for you. But on the six-week Fast Beach Diet, you should aim to step up the programme by experimenting with extensions to the original plan. These are suggestions not imperatives – so read, absorb and, if it feels right, have a go.

Try 4:3
One clear way to accelerate your Fast Diet is to add a third Fast Day each week for six weeks. In practice, this amounts to Alternate Day Fasting (ADF), and is the IF method that

has been most extensively investigated by researchers. To inspire you on your way, consider the following:

• A surprising finding during ADF trials was that people, when allowed to feast on a normal day, did not tend to do so. They reported not feeling particularly hungry after a day of fasting and rarely ate more than 110% of their normal calories[2]

• Another intriguing finding was that people on this form of IF lost more body fat than those doing a conventional calorie-restricting regime. If you go on a standard, medically approved diet (ie restricting your calorie intake every day) you will lose around 75% of weight as fat, 25% as muscle. On ADF, by contrast, the weight lost is almost entirely fat

What is also encouraging is that studies done with volunteers who have tried ADF show that those who stick to it report increasing feelings of fullness and dietary satisfaction over time. One explanation for this is that your stomach will shrink. So by all means give ADF or 4:3 a go. If it appeals, try it for six weeks only, always ensuring that you are meeting your nutritional needs over the course of a week – so, plenty of plants, adequate protein, occasional dairy, some 'good fats'. There's plenty of motivation and support later in this chapter.

Try 2-to-2

Some fasters get quite exercised about the precise timing of a fast. Michael and I are not overly prescriptive on this point:

our aim is to present a flexible plan that can be adapted to suit your own particular lifestyle and daily agenda. That said, it's clear that you can experiment with timing in order to maximise the effectiveness of a fast. You may, for instance, choose to fast, not from bedtime to bedtime, but from 2pm until 2pm, with reduced calories (or no calories) consumed at all during that 24-hour period. This is the method proposed by Canadian Brad Pilon in his seminal e-book *Eat Stop Eat* (if you haven't read it, I urge you to, particularly if you are interested in fitness and muscle mass).

If you choose to try the 2-to-2, here's how to go about it: after a normal lunch on Day 1, eat sparingly (or, if you follow Pilon's approach, nothing at all) until a late lunch the following day. That way, you fast as you sleep and no single day feels uncomfortably deprived of food. It's a clever trick, but it does require a modicum more concentration and commitment than the expressly straightforward whole-day option with its 500/600-calorie allowance. You might also choose to fast from supper to supper, which again means that no day is All Fast and No Fun. The point is that this plan is 'adjust to fit'. During the Fast Beach Diet, you may want to try a 2-to-2 full 24-hour fast to discover whether it's a good method for you. Stay playful, stay alert. Remember, you are in the driving seat, your foot poised delicately on the gas: if it feels wrong, pull over and revert to your usual 5:2 approach.

Extend your Fasting Window

Alternatively, you may simply choose to extend your normal Fasting Window. In the classic Fast Diet, we recommend breakfast, perhaps at 7am, then supper around 12 hours later. It's what works for me, and for many women who need a little sustenance to get the day going. This gives us 12 hours without food. However, as we know, plenty of successful Fast Dieters prefer to ignore breakfast entirely; these people – and I've found them to be mostly men – are effectively fasting for longer: from supper the previous night to supper on a Fast Day. On this regime, the Fasting Window can be as long as 24 hours – as with the 2-to2. This is something you may decide to try during the Fast Beach Diet. Perhaps give it a go for one of your weekly Fast Days. Remember, this is Fast Diet Plus, and it may not be to everyone's taste or benefit. Keep an open mind, stay strong, but always shut down a fast if it feels overwhelming.

Be fast-idious about your calorie quota

If you have been on the Fast Diet – or indeed, any diet – for a while, it's human instinct to develop a more blasé approach: you feel you know what's what, so you start to slip and an 'unconscious non-compliance' creeps in. While 5:2 demands that you 'comply' for only two days a week, it is still something of a challenge to apply yourself, to measure and count on those days. It is, as one 5:2 adherent says, 'a bit of a chore. And we humans are very good at avoiding chores.' For the next six weeks, don't guestimate, don't cheat, don't avoid the chore. Be particular. On Fast Days, renew your vows and be resolute about those calorie quotas. Apps such as MyFitnessPal will help you discover the calorie count of any given food.

Toughen up on non-Fast Days

You'll remember that the advice in *The Fast Diet* is to 'eat well for five days and reduce your calories for two'. It's the foundation of the 5:2 approach, but 'eating well' remains quite a vague proposition. The general thrust is that you shouldn't dwell upon calorie-counting on the five days a week when you're not fasting. But now, on the six-week Fast Beach Diet, we're going to toughen up on the non-Fast Days. For a short, contained period, it's time to really eat *well*. This will require some behavioural change, both subtle and direct. Again, you may choose to implement all of the suggestions in the pages ahead, or hand-pick those that best suit you. The idea here is to make some short-term sacrifices to get yourself beach-ready for summer. First up? The tricky subject of booze…

Cut out alcohol

I've put this first as it is the most effective way I know to kick-start the Fast Diet. I'm not expecting you to give up alcohol for ever, just for six short weeks. There are fantastically good reasons for doing so – and they're not all about weight loss.

If you're not sure how much good it will do you, a little experiment[3] performed in the offices of the *New Scientist* may be enough to get you on the wagon. On 5 October 2013, 14 members of the magazine's staff – all of whom considered themselves to be 'normal' drinkers – were given a range of tests to gauge the state of their livers and overall health. For the next five weeks, 10 of them drank no alcohol, while the other four continued as normal. Just over a month later, they returned to repeat the tests. For the four drinkers, there had been no significant changes. But in the abstainers, the impact had been dramatic. Their levels of liver fat – a precursor to liver damage – had fallen by an average of 15%. Their blood glucose levels had fallen a staggering 23% from 5.1 to 4.3mmol/l (the normal range is 3.9-5.6). They'd lost weight – 1.5kg on average. And their total blood cholesterol, a risk factor for heart disease, had dropped on average by 5%, from 4.6 to 4.4 mmo/l (a healthy level is anything below 5.2 mmo/l). The abstainers also reported sleeping better (up to 10% on the scale), and having improved concentration.

As the *New Scientist* went on to report in its January 2014 issue, Kevin Moore, a consultant in liver services at University College London Medical School, declared himself amazed by the results. 'What you have is a pretty average group of people who would not consider themselves heavy drinkers, yet stopping drinking *for a month* [my italics] alters liver fat, cholesterol and blood sugar and helps them lose weight. If someone did that with a health product, they'd be raking it in.'

If that's not quite enough to convince you, here are six more very good reasons to decline the wine for a brief period in order to jump-start your Fast Diet:

• Alcohol is chemically similar to sugar, so drinking it will set off the same insulin resistance that can promote weight gain

• It is stacked with calories and largely devoid of any

nutritional benefit. A recent survey[4] found that 85% of consumers don't know how many calories are in a glass of wine, and 63% don't consider wine when counting their calorie intake. But a 250ml glass of wine contains around 180 calories, a similar number to an ice cream; and remember – the higher the alcohol content, the more calories you're getting (see box below)

• Drink inhibits sleep (find out why this isn't great for weight loss on pages 62-64)

• It also stimulates appetite

• Nutritionists recognise that the body processes alcohol before it gets to work on fats and carbs – which means that drinking slows down the burning of fat for energy

In short, if you're really serious about trying to lose weight and gain health, consider a complete ban on alcohol for the duration of your FBD. You can always tuck into the sangria once you're on holiday.

CAN'T REJECT? THEN REDUCE

If you simply want to drink in a more controlled way during your six-week Fast Beach Diet, a few subtle changes can really cut your calorie count:
• Only ever half fill your glass
• Make every second drink water

• Keep the opened wine bottle in the fridge or cupboard, not on the table, where it's easier to reach for a refill
• Swap white wine for spritzers
• Keep adding ice cubes
• Choose small glasses (a 'glass of wine' used to be one unit; now – thanks to more generous glass sizes – it's two). And do be aware of visual illusions: research shows that people pour 28% more into short, wide glasses than tall ones[5]
• Watch your mixers. Soda water, lemon and lime juice are the best bet; orange juice will double the calorie count of a vodka shot
• Choose at least one night a week when you give alcohol a miss

THE CALORIES IN YOUR GLASS

Alcohol has around seven calories per gram, nearly twice that of protein or carbs, and is almost as calorific as fat. Brands and serving sizes will differ, but the following list gives a rough idea of the average calories in your drink.

Drink	Serving size	Calories
Bitter	1 pint (568ml)	180
Lager	1 pint (568ml)	150-240

Champagne	1 glass (120ml)	90
White wine	1 glass (120ml)	85
Red wine	1 glass (120ml)	80
Shot of gin	25ml	55
Shot of vodka	25ml	55
Whisky	25ml	55
Rum & Diet Coke	275ml	55
Glass of Baileys	37ml	120
Red Bull	250ml	110
Orange juice	250ml	115
Lemon juice	1 tbsp	4
Lime juice	1 tbsp	4

Shift your eating on non-Fast Days

So, for six weeks only, you'll need to watch what you eat on non-Fast Days as well as Fast Days and exert a degree of dietary restraint; the good news is that even modest changes in the way that you eat and the way that you think, can really make a difference.

Here's your best bet for success on the Fast Beach Diet:

• On a Fast Day, follow the 500/600-calorie rule

• On a non-Fast Day, eat healthily, moderately and with awareness

Simple, yes. But what does it mean in practice? On the Fast Beach Diet you do need to rethink a few attitudes, actions and habits in order to fulfil the 'eat healthily' part of the bargain. It's not a revolution. It's a recalibration, a time to reset your habits and expectations around food. Without assiduous calorie counting, it's now worth holding back on indulgences – the empty calories, extra helpings and superfluous snacks which may usually be part of your non-Fast Days.

The following are suggestions not edicts, a host of ideas for you to try, like a buffet of ways to introduce healthy eating into your life. Some may seem obvious, some you'll be doing already, others may steer you on a new course. The idea is to introduce as many healthy habits as possible over the course of your Fast Beach Diet, exercising just a bit more informed caution, a little more vigilance. So, pick and mix, remembering to keep it fairly simple and not so restrictive as to impact harshly upon your everyday life. This is not meant to be a punishment, and you shouldn't become a martyr to the cause. Here's how to accomplish the shift, realistically, positively and wisely.

Be far less refined
'People who eat white bread have no dreams!' proclaimed the great fashion editor Diana Vreeland – and, for some reason, her call to unrefined carbs has always stuck in my mind. One vital shift in thinking for Fast Beach Diet purposes is to recognise the difference between fast-acting and slow-acting carbohydrates.

For the next six weeks, focus on low-GI carbs which are slow-burning (jumbo oats, brown basmati rice, stone-ground wholemeal bread) rather than fast-burning (cake, crumpets, white bread). This is your best bet to bypass the sugar cycle – the familiar crave, consume, crash, crave, consume, crash spiral that we're keen to avoid during the Fast Beach Diet.

WHY INSULIN MATTERS

Highly refined carbs have a high GI so cause a spike in your blood-sugar levels, which then leads your pancreas to produce insulin. Insulin reduces the level of glucose in the bloodstream by diverting it to various body tissues for immediate use – or by storing it as fat. It also inhibits the conversion of body fat back into glucose for the body to burn. So insulin both facilitates the accumulation of fat, and then guards against its depletion. Insulin also acts on the brain to make you eat more, on your liver to manufacture more fat, and on the fat cells in your belly to store that fat. A steady blood-sugar level – encouraged by those slow-burn carbs which take time and energy to digest – will elicit a lower insulin response that can help to regulate your appetite. In other words, you're less likely to feel as hungry.

GETTING TO GRIPS WITH GI, GL AND IL

While I'd always recommend that you don't overthink

these things, it's worth having an eye on the blood-sugar impact of the foods you eat during your Fast Beach Diet.

As accustomed dieters will know, one way to discover which carbs cause a spike and which don't is to look at their Glycaemic Index (GI). Each food gets a score out of a 100 (pure sugar scores 100 on the GI scale). A low score means that the particular food does not tend to cause a rapid rise in blood glucose. These are the ones you want.

Of course, the size of the sugar spike depends not just on the food itself, but also on how much of it you eat. So there's also a measure called the Glycaemic Load:

$$\frac{GI \times grams\ of\ carbohydrate}{100}$$

You can find GI and GL scores for most carbs online. Do recognise that the numbers can be somewhat arbitrary and occasionally contradictory – so if you're keen to have precise numbers, perhaps take an average of several sources. Diabetes UK has an excellent guide at www.diabetes.org.uk.

More recently, nutritionists have started to turn their attention to the Insulin Load (IL) based on a given food's Insulin Index[6] – a number designed to reveal which foods give a surge of insulin by measuring the post-prandial increase in insulin secretion of a whole food, including the interactions between, say, carbs, proteins and fats. This is the crunch. What you really want to know on your Fast Beach Diet is which foods are likely to promote a lower insulin response than others. Porridge, for example, elicits a lower insulin response than muesli; milk has a higher than expected IL, as does beef. As a general rule of thumb, foods with a high Insulin Index include refined cereals, sweets, white bread and potatoes, while most vegetables – no surprise here – produce a negligible insulin response.

Cook at home

Three easy little words. But quite a tricky concept to work into everyday life if you're up to your neck in work and kids, and the ready-meal is right there, looking so very convenient in its plastic jacket and jazzy sleeve. I understand. Cooking from scratch doesn't always fit. But try to make time to cook, just for the next six weeks. If you can't do it daily, do it often. If you can't do it often, do it sometimes (in batches, then freeze it).

You may, of course, already be a kitchen connoisseur: now it's time to get those calorie counts down. Remember, home cooking means you can control the quality and the quantity of what you eat; besides, cooking in summertime really is a breeze – sometimes a simple question of opening the salad drawer and grabbing the chopping board (do ensure that your fridge can deliver; see pages 140-141 for a quick Fast-friendly shopping list). Check out chapter 7 for plenty of Fast Diet cooking tips and my new summer recipes – many of which take less time to prepare than it takes to undress a ready-meal and get it to go ping – or look at the hundreds of ideas in *The Fast Diet Recipe Book* and *Fast Cook*.

Cut back on treats

'Treats.' Remember those? An occasional pleasure. A rare delight. I don't want to get all misty-eyed and rose-tinted, but when I was a child, a treat was exactly that: a finger of fudge, a Custard Cream, two sherbet lemons, something you had sometimes, not always, when you'd been particularly good. These days, 'treats' are almost a food group in their own right. You only have to queue to pay at a petrol station to be engulfed in a roiling sea of snacks and grab bags and cookies and chocolate and STOP! Let's get some perspective here and put the treats back in their box. Not for ever. Just for a bit.

One of the pillars of the success of the Fast Diet is, of course, that it expressly allows occasional treats: it's what makes the regime sustainable and feasible over the long term. Alleluia. But during the Fast Beach Diet, it's time for tough love. Rather than eliminate, recalibrate. Remember, it's ONLY FOR SIX WEEKS (did I mention that?).

Packaging? Pack it in

One super-simple way to facilitate healthy eating is to gravitate towards foods with very little packaging: the ratio of plastic to foodstuff is generally a pretty good indication of its nutritional value. Products that don't require much in the way of packaging tend to feature fewer stabilisers, additives or E-numbers than their overly packaged cousins.

While following the Fast Beach Diet, also beware of 'low-fat' foods, where the fat has often simply been replaced with sugar. They have a 'health halo' effect that can actually encourage you to eat more (curiously, research has shown that low-fat labels lead people to eat 16-23% more calories in total)[7]. Similarly, don't fall for the seductive health claims on the packet. Words like 'wholesome' are largely puff, designed to make you feel good and fish out your purse. Better to read the back of the packet than the front.

Ban the big no-nos

The list of foods to avoid throughout the Fast Beach Diet will come as no surprise: packaged desserts, sweet fizzy drinks, commercial cereals and fast food should all be out of bounds for the next month and a half. But there's one killer combo that you really need to eliminate for as long as possible…

CUT THE 50:50S

Foods high in fat and sugar, as we all know, can be very appealing, but what has recently been discovered is that in combination they are *particularly* tempting; we crave this mix and we find it very difficult to stop eating it once we've got going. According to neuroscientist Professor Paul Kenny at the Scripps Research Institute in Florida, food with a 50:50 fat:sugar ratio interferes with our mechanisms of self-regulation[8]; there's simply no 'off' switch, as there would be when consuming either macronutrient alone. Scientists call this 'hedonic eating'. It supercharges the brain's reward system and overrides satiety signals. Interestingly, this particular 50:50 fat-sugar ratio doesn't happen in nature. But it does happen in cheesecake. And doughnuts. And those moist chocolate fudge cakes that look so fetching in supermarkets and coffee shops, the saucy sirens of the bakery world. So, make a commitment. No 50:50s for the duration of the Fast Beach Diet. None. I bet they'll look a lot less alluring after six weeks...

Go Mediterranean

One way to ensure that you eat healthily and wisely throughout your Fast Beach Diet is to stick to a Mediterranean diet on the five days a week when you're not fasting. 'Mediterranean' is a shorthand way of saying 'cut the junk and get real'. This approach will be familiar to anyone who has read Dr Michelle Harvie's *2-Day Diet*, based on her research at the Genesis Breast Cancer Prevention Centre. The idea is to follow a carefully defined and controlled diet for two consecutive days, and then stick to fruit, veg, wholegrains, pulses, nuts, olive oil, lean protein and unsweetened dairy on your five 'non-diet' days each week.

It is certainly an effective way to lose weight. In her studies Dr Harvie found that female dieters who stuck to her plan for 12 weeks lost an average of 6.4kg (1st) and 2 inches (5cm) from their waists and hips. Some did much better, losing as much as 14.5kg (2st 3lb) and dropping two dress sizes. So a six-week sabbatical in the Mediterranean? Why not?

Think summer, eat summer

Another way to sharpen up your eating habits at this time of year is simply, consciously, to embrace the season. As the days lengthen and the weather improves, it's easier – in fact, it's obvious – to shift to fewer carbs and fats, more salads and fresh veg. Here's how to go about it:

• **Change how you cook to suit summer:** simply going from fried to grilled and using a multi-level steamer will save significant calories on any day of the week

• **Roll out the barbecue:** it's one of the best low-cal ways to cook protein, whether it's slapped direct on the grill or wrapped in foil and tucked into the embers

• **Go raw:** the idea – if you want to stick to the method advocated by 'raw foodists' – is that nothing should be heated beyond 118°C (the point at which some vitamins are lost). During your Fast Beach Diet, consider introducing a raw day once a week (on a Fast or a Non-Fast Day). It's worth noting that some nutrients are less available in raw foods than cooked – the beta carotene in carrots, for example, or the lycopene in tomatoes. But a raw day is a great way to treat yourself to fresh tastes and a fresh approach, shaking up old-pattern eating habits. Try Pen's beetroot salad on page 130 for inspiration. Or – a startlingly simple suggestion – just eat more Japanese food. The Japanese have some of the lowest obesity rates in the developed world, in part because their diet contains a lot of food served in varying degrees of rawness

• **Go fish:** the Japanese also tend to consume a good deal less meat than Westerners. Fish are high in protein and some, such as salmon, mackerel and tuna – the oily fish – are also high in omega-3 essential fatty acids (though higher in calories too). Go for sashimi over sushi (that way, you avoid rice) for the perfect summer supper. For an Italian version of sashimi, try crudo: slice ultra-fresh raw fish – bass, bream or mackerel – into tissue-thin strips and serve dressed with a little olive oil, lemon and fresh herbs rather than the usual trio of Japanese accompaniments

A SIMPLE SUMMER CEVICHE

If you find completely raw fish a challenge, try ceviche, where acid in a citrus marinade 'cooks' the fish without heat. This is a traditional Latin American method – which also happens to be deeply fashionable in certain London postcodes at the moment (perhaps as a response to our newly acquired taste for low-carb food). Not surprisingly, it requires the freshest fish you can find.

Combine the juice of a lime and the juice of a

lemon with one finely diced red onion, one red chilli (deseeded and finely chopped, to taste), salt and pepper and a dash of Tabasco. Add a good handful of chopped coriander and a fillet of fresh fish, boned, skinned and cubed or sliced, per person. Place all the ingredients in a non-reactive bowl and refrigerate for half an hour, then serve.

Have soup before supper... or at any time

Soup, according to research from Penn State University,[9] is a great appetite suppressant because it consists of a hunger-busting combination of liquids and solids; eat it before a meal and you can lower your overall calorie intake by up to 20% compared to a meal without soup. So eat soup – winter warm or summer chilled – regularly during your six-week Fast Beach Diet. A light veggie broth is an ideal way to get water and fibre into your stomach to start to signal fullness before you embark on the meal proper.

On a non-Fast Day, consider replacing your usual lunch-time sandwich with a simple soup – just doing this will eliminate 10 slices of bread (and butter) from your weekly consumption. To keep the calories under control, choose veg-based broths rather than thick creamy or meaty soups, the kind you can stand your spoon up in. Me? I'm a sucker for pho, a Vietnamese broth packed with fresh herbs and chilli. Look out for it on your lunchtime takeaway menu, or make your own, following the recipe on page 134.

Implement the Rule of Three-Quarters

You want simple? Here's simple. Fill your plate with veg at the expense of meat and carbs – a 75:25 ratio would be ideal. This single, relatively small change can make a huge difference to your calorie and nutrient intake over the course of the six weeks.

It's no surprise to learn that we in the rich world eat three or four times as much animal protein as we need, and most of the nutrients we get from our meat-mania are just as available from plants (150g of nuts and seeds a day will do the job).

While meat is generally a good source of protein and certain micronutrients, it can be high in saturated fat and cholesterol. Studies have found that a vegan or vegetarian diet can be highly effective for weight loss[10], and vegetarian populations tend to have lower rates of heart disease, high blood pressure, diabetes and obesity[11].

Even if wholesale vegetarianism isn't on your agenda, cutting back on red and processed meat consumption certainly makes sense on any number of levels – at least for the duration of your Fast Beach Diet. So how else can you start the shift?

• Institute a meat-free day each week – a Meatless Monday, perhaps. Or go further and stay meat-free all week, with meat reserved for a weekend treat

• Avoid the 'meat as main course' mentality; think Veg First. Give plants a starring role on your plate, not a bit part

• Cook plants as you would meat – roast, grill, griddle, bake – to give them that central function

There's another, perhaps more pedestrian, advantage to increasing the vegetable content of your meals, and it has to do with bulk. Eating 'big' foods containing plenty of fibre and water – loads of leaves, stacks of salad, great piles of greens – will fill you up for fewer calories. That's what you want in the weeks ahead.

A QUICK WORD ON VITAMIN C

Fibre. Nutrients. Volume. Yes, you already know eating plenty of veg makes sense. What you may not know is that vitamin C, among its many health benefits, may well be crucial for weight management. According to researchers from Arizona State University, individuals who consume an adequate amount of vitamin C burn 30% more fat during moderate exercise than those who don't get enough of the stuff[12]. They also showed that too little vitamin C in the bloodstream correlates with increased body fat and waist measurements. Remember that vitamin C is easily lost – so if you're cooking leafy veg, do it quickly. Steaming is ideal.

Watch what you drink

We've already talked about limiting your alcohol intake while on the Fast Beach Diet; but there are equally good reasons for cutting back on soft drinks too. While many of us are aware of the calories loaded on our forks, the ones that lurk in cups and glasses frequently go uncounted. You may well need to modify your behaviour, so make the commitment, write it down and have alternatives to hand. As you'll discover later in this chapter, with recognition and repetition, habits can be modified. After six weeks, your daily caramel latte will seem about as appealing as a triple-layer cream cake with cream on the side.

First, junk the juice

Beware the 'health halo' of smoothies and juices. Fruit juice is ultimately a higher-sugar, lower-fibre version of its source. Juicing eliminates the skins of the fruits, precisely where most of their health-giving flavonoids and carotenoids are concentrated; the skins are also the primary source of fibre – important for the health of your gut, and useful in slowing down the digestion and absorption of the juice's sugars.

Commercial smoothies can have a similar sugar content to Coke and, because they are acidic, they are corrosive to your teeth; they are also loaded with calories. Have an apple instead, or choose one of the drinks in the Fast-friendly list on pages 60-61.

If you are thinking about trying veg juices as an alternative, be aware that carrot and tomato juice are at the higher end of the calorie spectrum, while green veg juice is at the lower end.

THE GREEN GREEN JUICE OF HOME

Trendy? Yes. Faddish? Possibly. But green juices do have substantial nutritional value, and significantly less sugar than their fruit equivalents. They usually involve great gusts of leafy veg and brassicas such as kale, spinach, chard or broccoli – far more than you could possibly consume in a single sitting. The dark green veg contain a glorious cargo of vitamins and minerals – so it's little wonder that many fasters swear by them to start the day, and all for wonderfully few calories. You may like to try some of these favourite combinations:

• Kale, mint and apple
• Spinach, spring greens, cavolo nero, apple and lemon juice
• Watercress, parsley, cucumber and ginger
• Romaine lettuce, celery and green pear
• Rocket, spinach, pear and lime

But a few rules of thumb:

• Don't store it; drink green juice immediately as it degrades quickly
• You'll be getting the vitamins and minerals of your chosen veg, but far less of their soluble fibre – which is the really good stuff for your cholesterol and blood pressure
• Your best bet is a fresh green juice rather than a bottled one, which will almost certainly have been pasteurised – great for its shelf life, but not

for its nutritional value
- Be careful with green juices if you are on anti-depressants or blood-thinning meds

No pop... sorry, not even Diet Coke

Most fasters will have already eliminated 'full-fat' fizzy drinks from their repertoire on a Fast Day, knowing that they're liquid calorie traps. Good reasons, then, to drop the pop for the duration of the Fast Beach Diet on non-Fast Days too. You can do it. We can help. Look at the list below for dozens of no-cal and lo-cal drinks, with a particular emphasis on delicious and unusual summertime tastes.

But what about the tricky question of diet fizz? I know that lots of Fast Diet fans rely on a Diet Coke to get them through to supper with their temper intact. But, listen up: counter-intuitive as it may seem, some studies suggest that consuming zero-calorie sweeteners *increases* the risk of putting on weight[13]. Scientists at Purdue University in Indiana analysed the link and found that rats fed yoghurt sweetened with saccharin (a sugar substitute) ate more, and grew fatter, than those eating yoghurt sweetened with glucose (the real thing). The researchers submitted that sweet foods provide an 'orosensory stimulus' that convinces the body that a deluge of calories is on its way. When, as with diet drinks, the advertised calories don't materialise, the system becomes confused – and as a result 'people eat more or expend less energy than they otherwise would'.

Even if you're not convinced by this line of reasoning, what's indisputable is that the makers of processed diet foods and drinks tend to replace fats and sugars with synthetic alternatives and 'lab-designed' compounds. During the Fast Beach Diet, try to wean yourself off the fake foods like these. Again, habit can be a surprisingly fragile beast: fight it for a while and it will almost certainly disappear, like a shadow when you turn on the light.

Choose your coffee carefully

There's a growing body of evidence to suggest that, far from being a guilty pleasure, coffee may be good for you, helping to prevent mental decline, improve cardiac health and reduce the risk of diabetes, liver cancer and stroke[14]. It does matter, however, what you order from your friendly local barista. A Starbucks grande whole milk caffé mocha with whipped cream, to take one ridiculous example, has 396 calories. Even a Costa caffé latte with skimmed has 71. And a double espresso? Just 11. So, decide right now to ditch the gaudy coffees that have danced into our lives and taken up lazy residence. Try instead, just for this six weeks, to drink your coffee black and sugarless. If you still despise it after several attempts, have just a dash of milk to take the edge off. Remember: the Fast Beach Diet is a short, sharp wake-up call, and for the next six weeks you do need to stay gently alert, like a seated (not sleeping) guard at the gate.

WHAT TO DRINK IN SUMMERTIME

- Vanilla tea – hot or chilled. Add a slice or two of fresh root ginger
- Coconut water – a good alternative to sports

---

drinks, it's natural and low in sugar (it still has 83 calories per 330ml carton, though, so go easy)

• If tap water doesn't turn you on, buy a water filter and keep a jug of filtered water in the fridge, perhaps with added slices of lemon, lime, mint, lemongrass, basil leaves or cucumber

• Chilled herbal tea – try peppermint tea over ice with crushed fresh mint leaves. Iced cranberry and pomegranate tea are great too – keep them in the fridge and serve with slices of fresh orange

• Hot water with lemon and ginger; or with cloves, lemongrass or even a slice of red chilli

• Green tea – plenty of people believe in the fat-busting, antioxidant power of green tea. But all you really need to absorb is that it has virtually no calories, and about half the caffeine of coffee.

• The same goes for Chinese pu-er tea, which comes in cake form, to be crumbled into boiling water. Devotees speak of its capacity to reduce cholesterol and raise the metabolic rate; again, the jury's out – but if you enjoy it, dive right in

• Virgin mojito, made with soda, mint, lime and a bruised lemongrass stalk to stir. Serve on the rocks in a tall glass

• Home-made lemon iced tea – make a tea of your choice (English breakfast can't be beaten), chill, add lemon or orange slices, or a squeeze of juice and thin tendrils of the zest. Add a teaspoon of agave if you need a little sweetener

- No-added sugar cordials – make it dilute – with still or sparkling water. Freeze diluted elderflower cordials into lollies or cubes to have on hot days
- Iced black coffee – simply pour espresso over ice cubes and sip
- At bedtime, if sleep is elusive, try warm skimmed milk with nutmeg, a dash of vanilla essence and a cinnamon stick to stir

Sleep well

There are dozens of published research papers that link poor sleep with weight gain. Researchers at the University of Warwick analysed the relationship between sleep and obesity[15] and found that that adults who slept for fewer than five hours a night were one and a half times more likely to be obese. Why?

The answer comes from studies of leptin and ghrelin, two of the hormones that govern appetite. For some reason, I think of them as characters from *The Lord of the Rings* – leptin, the elf that keeps the hypothalamus informed about the adequacy of your energy stores, is the satiety hormone that suppresses appetite; and ghrelin is the belly dwarf whose job it is to signal hunger to the brain.

Leptin, secreted by fat cells, has a circadian rhythm and reaches its peak during sleep. If you're not sleeping well, peak leptin levels are not reached and the brain sends out its minions – hunger pangs and energy conservation. At the same time, lack of sleep causes ghrelin levels to rise. Your appetite kicks in and calorie-dense, dopamine-generating snacks become irresistible.

There have been innumerable investigations– sometimes resulting in hyperbolic claims – into sleep and its effect on leptin and ghrelin. A swift round-up might include:

• A study[16] of 1000 volunteers at Stanford University found that those who slept fewer than eight hours a night had lower levels of leptin and higher levels of ghrelin, and they also had higher levels of body fat. 'Specifically, those who slept the fewest hours per night weighed the most'

• Researchers at Bristol University[17] compared blood samples from insomniacs and good sleepers. The former had leptin levels 15% below normal, and ghrelin levels 15% above normal

• A study at Laval University in Quebec[18] found that there may be an ideal 'sleep zone' of around eight hours a night that facilitates body-weight regulation

None of this is incontrovertible evidence that a good night's sleep will encourage fat loss on your Fast Beach Diet. But it is worth knowing that sleep is far from a passive state; disrupt it and our bodies will inevitably suffer. Besides, whatever our hormones are doing, poor sleep will certainly rob us of the energy required to bounce out of bed and make the best of a day. This low-energy cycle is the enemy of sustainable weight loss, since sugary, salty, starchy snacks are incomparably more enticing when we're tired.

So, commit to going to bed at a reasonable time while on your diet. Try and get a decent eight-hour sleep every night for the next six weeks (much easier, incidentally, when you go alcohol-free). It will do you the world of good, and may even help shift those scales.

HOW TO GET YOUR ZZZZS WITH EASE

- Institute a screen ban: no screens, no tablets, no phones at bedtime. If your bedroom looks like the control room at NASA, unplug it now
- Get up at a regular time: no matter when you went to sleep, rise at the same time each day. This helps to programme your body clock into a good sleep-wake pattern, which can be hugely helpful for insomniacs
- Nap with care: if you're feeling done in by mid-afternoon, take just a short 15-minute nap. Beyond that, you'll eat into your body's sleep needs and may disrupt your night

Tune in on any day

You'll have already absorbed that 5:2 is a limited but effective discipline; what it requires is a change of behaviour. A change of mind. Part of its intention (and one of the prime reasons for its success) is that it encourages you to be observant, 'mindful', around food – certainly on your two Fast Days. On the Fast Beach Diet, you need to be that much more aware, for that much more of the time. This needn't be a burden; it can be a fascinating undertaking that serves to illuminate entrenched behaviour around food and eating.

In addition, it's important to get a handle on habit, on temptation and on cravings – the trio of trips that can up-end you on the fast track to weight loss and good health. It's time to retrain your brain.

Cultivate mindfulness around food

Mindfulness is a fashionable concept these days, but it is rooted in age-old wisdom that can, and should, affect your relationship with everything in your world, including calories. The key is to live consciously. I'm keen on a quote from Henry Miller, who said that 'the aim of life is to live, and to live means to be aware, joyously, drunkenly, serenely, divinely aware'. Sounds gorgeous, right? But what does it mean in practice, particularly with regard to the food on your plate? Here are my tips for mindful eating:

• **Don't eat on auto-pilot**. Throughout the diet, eat with awareness, allowing yourself to absorb the fascinating fact that you're eating. Don't eat on the way to doing something else. Don't read, watch TV, text, Facebook, drive or juggle at the same time. Tune into the food on your fork. Look at it. Really taste it. That way, you'll enjoy each mouthful. You'll also know when you've had enough. On non-Fast Days, stay alert. Eat until you're satisfied, not until you're full (this will come naturally after a few weeks' practice)

• **Slow down**. It seems a simple enough suggestion, but just think about how often you bolt your food. For the duration of your Fast Beach Diet, sit to eat. Stay put in one place. Make it an event. Eat at a table. Drink a glass of water first. Say grace, if that's your thing. Anything to make you tune in. Eat with intent. Put down your knife and fork between bites. Let your body know what's just hit it, recognising that it takes your stomach a few minutes to catch up with your mouth; wait 10 minutes before that extra spoonful. Wait again before embarking on pudding. You may not need it today

• **Guard against portion distortion**. This is the thinking that convinces us that the food piled on our plates – or the amount that is given to us in a 'serving' – is the quantity we really want and need. It's a habit, nothing more. So break it. Learn when to say 'when'. Have a care for the amount of food you're putting on your plate at every meal. Bear in mind that a person will eat an average of 92% of any food they serve themselves[19]. So, for the next six weeks, serve a bit less.

Be particularly aware when ordering food when you're out. Portion sizes have rocketed over the last 20 years – compare a modern cupcake to the fairy cakes of your childhood – thanks in part to the availability of cheap food and the canny commercial practices of the food industry. But we humans are prone to a behaviour that psychologists call 'unit bias': if the food is moderately palatable, we'll go on eating the amount that's put in front of us until it's gone; we also tend to eat more when offered more[20]. Once you absorb this, you'll realise you really can put the brakes on

• **Give yourself visual clues**. Yes, smaller plates can be a startlingly effective way to limit your eating (studies have shown that moving from a 12-inch to a 10-inch dinner plate leads people to serve and eat 22% less)[21]; dark plates are also thought to be helpfuzl, since you can more clearly discern the amount of food in front of you

• **Wait before you eat**. Don't eat as soon as the clock says 'lunchtime'. If you feel hungry during a Fast Day – or on a non-Fast Day during the next six weeks – try to resist for at least 10 minutes to see whether the hunger subsides (as it naturally tends to do). The idea is to put food in its place. It's only food. Once you start to think about food in a rational and realistic way, you'll discover that you can modify your behaviour around it. You can even playfully push it aside. You may discover, as many fasters attest, that you develop a keen sensitivity to your own appetite, hunger and satiety. These will change from day to day. Stay quiet, and you can begin to feel these subtle, visceral things. In time – and six weeks is enough time – you'll learn to turn the dial this way or that, up or down, depending on your needs on any given day

• **Keep a food diary**. Dieters who keep food diaries are known to be more successful at losing weight than those who don't, with one study[22] finding that it can double weight loss as part of a managed programme. Logging one's consumption seems to heighten awareness; the simple act of quantifying incoming food (and, don't forget, drink) seems to be enough to still your hand as it wanders towards the biscuits. During the Fast Beach Diet, catalogue your intake on Fast Days and non-Fast Days, using the planner included in this book.

Temptation, habit and cravings: how to negotiate the hurdles ahead

On average, we make 227 food-related decisions every day (most people, when questioned, wildly underestimate the number and guess that it's about 14)[23]. That's plenty of choice, and plenty of opportunities to fall face down into the nearest custard tart.

On a diet, most of us are subject to what social psychologists call 'dynamic inconsistency' – we tumble into the gap between what we plan in good faith and what we do in real time. And what usually gets in the way or leads us astray is a potent cocktail of temptation, habit and the collapse of willpower in the face of cravings.

Tackling temptation

Your mission for the next six weeks, and perhaps beyond, is to recognise temptation for what it is. Temporal. Transient. Fleeting and ephemeral. It is also particular to you. While there are universal experiences, temptation – like love and death – is intensely personal; your job is to unravel what makes you succumb, then try and avert and subvert it. And there are plenty of acknowledged ways to do this:

• **Act upon the Proximity Principle** and put temptation out of reach. One study (using Hershey's Kisses) showed how having food conveniently close makes you eat a great deal more of it[24]. When workers kept the chocolate on their desk, they ate an average of nine Kisses per day; when it was moved just six feet away, they ate only four per day. So, for the next six weeks, remove temptation. Don't give yourself the choice of whether to eat the Kettle Chips or not; don't put the Kettle Chips on the table. Better yet, don't buy them

• **Conversely, make healthy food abundantly available.** Have it to hand. At mealtimes, serve vegetables and salads in help-yourself bowls on the dining table – but serve meat, cheese, bread, pasta, potatoes and pudding away from the table to prevent the idle digging-in of a finger or a fork

• **Just cook enough.** Not too much, but just enough, remembering that leftovers are somehow all the more delicious for being left over

• **For the next six weeks, don't eat straight from a box**, bag, carton or tub. Serve yourself a bowl of – whatever – and then put the carton away. Research has also shown that people eat more when given a larger container of food than when they're given a smaller container[25]. So think petite

• **Don't get side-tracked.** It's worth noting that if you are distracted, you are more likely to give into temptation; in one study, students trying to remember a telephone number were 50% more likely to choose chocolate cake over fruit from a snack trolley[26]. When your mind is preoccupied, it makes impulsive, 'primitive brain' choices based on urges and instincts; this sits nicely with our ideas about mindful eating. Your job is to tune in and choose right

• **Your goal must outweigh your temptation.** This may seem obvious (otherwise, you'd never get going). But you need reminding, at the very instant that your hand gravitates towards the bread bin and the butter knife. So try site-specific aversion therapy. If necessary, tape a picture of yourself – the selfie you'd never post on Facebook, the holiday snap that made you embark on the Fast Diet in the first place – to the fridge door. Simple and aggressive, but effective

Habits: how to make them, how to break them

Our mission on the Fast Beach Diet is to find ways to happily abstain in a world of incomparable abundance. As Aristotle said, 'we are what we repeatedly do'; it's time now to dismantle poor habits and install the good. Popular thinking has it (probably erroneously) that it takes just 21 days to make or break a habit – the truth, however, is that the timing depends largely on what that habit is, and who's doing it. One study at University College London[27] found that it took 66 days to adopt the habit of eating fruit daily, while the habit of drinking a glass of water after breakfast took just 20 days to install. The important thing is to repeat, and repeat, and repeat. As the study (and Aristotle) said, 'with repetition of a behaviour in a consistent context, automaticity increases'. That's what you want. This is subtle stuff – a call to rewire your brain. Here's how to go about it...

• **Change the record.** A study has revealed that up to 45% of what we do every day is habitual[28] – performed without thinking in the same place at the same time in the same bovine way. We respond, automatically, to outside stimuli. Acting without thinking is a central driver of habits. Think about checking your emails. Fancying a coffee. Where you sit to watch TV. The route you take on your bike to work. 'Habits are formed when the memory associates specific actions with specific places or moods,' Professor Wendy Wood of Duke University in North Carolina told the *New York Times*. 'If you regularly eat chips while sitting on the couch, after a while, seeing the couch will automatically prompt you to reach for the Doritos.'

Your mission for the next six weeks is to undermine your instinctive bias for the status quo. Turn left when you usually turn right. Sit on a different seat on the Tube. Take the stairs, not the lift. When you experience a compulsion to eat too much, or to eat badly, it's time to face it head on. You are a rational being and you are making a specific, time-sensitive decision to eat that cheeseburger or pour that glass of wine. You really do have the power to choose, at each incremental, individual moment. Once you recognise this power, it is possible to overcome the cognitive bias that leads to impulsive snacking and compulsive eating. Try to install a behaviour – not for ever, just for this precise moment – which alters your established route. This is called 'deliberate practice'; it takes grit and determination. Leave the table. Stretch your legs. Don't eat in front of the TV (chuck out the tray that makes it possible). Change the picture

• **Be specific**. Research shows that vague plans are more likely to fail – so avoid abstraction, waffle and generalisations. Think through exactly what you are going to do, where you are going to do it, and at what time. For example, instead of saying that you will go running two days a week, tell yourself that you will run on Sundays and Wednesdays at 7pm. Instead of saying 'I'll cut back on treats' say 'I won't have my morning muffin'. Similarly, as we've established above, if you want to lose weight, there is a psychological advantage in setting a specific goal for how much weight (10lb?), by when (15th August when you fly to Majorca?)

• **Think carrots not sticks**. A study from the University of Chicago[29] outlines how positive feedback on new habits will increase the likelihood of success. Don't be afraid to recognise and grandstand your achievements. Website forums make an ideal platform for a bit of back-patting – go to www.thefastdiet.co.uk to find tons of support and praise in action. Plenty of people on our site say that this is often enough to get them through a tricky patch

• **Decode your brain**. Appetite is governed by a complex interaction of hormones, neurotransmitters and enzymes – and we don't have a clear picture of the precise interrelations at work as we eat, or as we fast. What we do know is that hunger has a biochemical basis: grasping just a little about what your hormones are up to can really help when you're attempting to change habits or overcome temptation. Let's return to leptin, the satiety hormone which encourages you to stop eating when you're full. Its message can be

the
fast beach
diet DAY BY DAY PLANNER

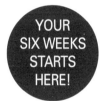

YOUR SIX WEEKS STARTS HERE!

Mark out your Fast Days on the chart for the next six weeks – perhaps get yourself a neon highlighter pen to plot the course ahead. Make sure that your diary can accommodate a fast on those days. Clear the decks and make sure you have Fast-friendly food to hand.

Make a note of your starting stats. Measure your start weight – be honest – and your target weight – be realistic. Measure your start BMI and your initial fitness. Tell your family and friends you're doing it. Tell yourself you can do it. Six weeks will disappear in the blink of an eye.

Start weight

Target weight

Start BMI

To measure this, go to thefastdiet.co.uk or download the new Fast Beach Diet app

Strength test: number of push-ups

Anybody who finds it hard to do standard push-ups can do modified push-ups, ie resting on your elbows rather than on your hands

Fat %

The easiest way to do this is with weighing scales that measure your fat percentage as well as your weight

Resting heart rate

This is to measure your cardio fitness: either use a gadget, or take your pulse for 10 seconds and multiply the result by 6 to get your heart rate per minute

week 1

WHAT TO EXPECT If you've never fasted before, the first Fast Day can be tough. Keep busy. Stay hydrated. Your mission is simple: get through the day, reminding yourself that tomorrow will be easier. Remember, hunger will pass.

Food diary

Date	Fast Day?	Calories eat	Calories from drinks
1			
2			
3			
4			
5			
6			
7			

Weigh-in after Fast Day 1

Weigh-in after Fast Day 2

Waist measurement day 7

BMI day 7

Fat % day 7

Exercise diary

Date	Cardio completed	Strength training
1		
2		
3		
4		
5		
6		
7		

Strength test day 7

Resting heart rate day 7

How are you feeling?

week 2

WHAT TO EXPECT You've knocked off two full-on Fast Days and know the ropes
now. Stay focused. Your Fast Days should start getting easier from now on.

Food diary

Date	Fast Day?	Calories eat	Calories from drinks
1			
2			
3			
4			
5			
6			
7			

Weigh-in after Fast Day 1 _____   Waist measurement day 7 _____   Fat %
                                                                                 day 7
Weigh-in after Fast Day 2 _____   BMI day 7 _____   _____

Exercise diary

Date	Cardio completed	Strength training
1		
2		
3		
4		
5		
6		
7		

Strength test day 7 _____   How are you feeling? _____

Resting heart rate day 7 _____   _____

week 3

'If we are facing in the right direction, all we have to do is keep on walking'
Buddhist saying

WHAT TO EXPECT By the end of this week, you'll be halfway through, so take heart. If you're seeing movement on the scales, use that to bounce you through these middle weeks. As your fitness increases, step up your HIT by increasing resistance or reps.

Food diary

Date	Fast Day?	Calories eat	Calories from drinks
1			
2			
3			
4			
5			
6			
7			

Weigh-in after Fast Day 1 _____   Waist measurement day 7 _____   Fat % day 7

Weigh-in after Fast Day 2 _____   BMI day 7 _____

Exercise diary

Date	Cardio completed	Strength training
1		
2		
3		
4		
5		
6		
7		

Strength test day 7 _____   How are you feeling?

Resting heart rate day 7 _____

week 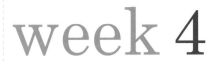 4

*'Don't dig your grave with
your own knife and fork'*
English proverb

WHAT TO EXPECT New habits are beginning to form. Congratulate yourself,
reward yourself and tell people about your achievements. If you're feeling a bit
lost, go on the forums (ours is at www.thefastdiet.co.uk) for support, advice and
a group hug.

Food diary

Date	Fast Day?	Calories eat	Calories from drinks
1			
2			
3			
4			
5			
6			
7			

Weigh-in after Fast Day 1 _____

Weigh-in after Fast Day 2 _____

Waist measurement day 7 _____

BMI day 7 _____

Fat %
day 7

_____

Exercise diary

Date	Cardio completed	Strength training
1		
2		
3		
4		
5		
6		
7		

Strength test day 7 _____

Resting heart rate day 7 _____

How are you feeling? _____

_____

week 5

'Success is a staircase, not a doorway'
Dottie Walters

WHAT TO EXPECT You've been doing the FB Diet for over a month now, and you may find that your appetite and taste for food has started to change. Check your portion sizes: have they got smaller? If you've managed without alcohol, your body will have started to gain measurable benefit. Not long now till you can celebrate…

Food diary

Date	Fast Day?	Calories eat	Calories from drinks
1			
2			
3			
4			
5			
6			
7			

Weigh-in after Fast Day 1 _____   Waist measurement day 7 _____   Fat % day 7

Weigh-in after Fast Day 2 _____   BMI day 7 _____

Exercise diary

Date	Cardio completed	Strength training
1		
2		
3		
4		
5		
6		
7		

Strength test day 7 _____   How are you feeling? _____

Resting heart rate day 7 _____

week 6

'When you reach the end of your rope, tie a knot in it and hang on'
Thomas Jefferson

WHAT TO EXPECT The final week of the Fast Beach Diet: the habits and techniques you're installing now will help you in the days ahead as you resume your 5:2. Occasional treats will be back on the menu. Just one more week of tough love and you're done.

Food diary

Date	Fast Day?	Calories eat	Calories from drinks
1			
2			
3			
4			
5			
6			
7			

Weigh-in after Fast Day 1

Weigh-in after Fast Day 2

Waist measurement day 7

BMI day 7

Fat % day 7

Exercise diary

Date	Cardio completed	Strength training
1		
2		
3		
4		
5		
6		
7		

Strength test day 7

Resting heart rate day 7

Congratulations! You should be feeling great...

The Fast Beach Diet checklist

Tighten up on Fast Days
Go to 4:3
Try 2-to-2
Extend your Fasting Window
Be fast-idious about your Fast Day calorie quota

Toughen up on non-Fast Days
Cut out alcohol
Or reduce alcohol intake
Shift your eating habits
Avoid refined carbs
Cook at home when you can
Cut back on treats
Choose unpackaged food
Cut the 50/50s
Move towards a Mediterranean diet
Cook to suit the summertime
    Grill and barbecue
    Choose raw foods
    Embrace Japanese food
    Eat more fish
    Choose soup
    Implement the Rule of Three-Quarters
    Have a Meatless Monday
    Go demi-vegi and make meat a once-a-week treat
Watch what you drink
Junk the juice
Drop the pop
Choose the right coffee
Sleep well
Get a good eight hours in

Tune in on any day
Cultivate mindfulness around food
Don't eat on auto-pilot
Stop when you're satisfied, not when you're full
Give yourself visual clues
Smaller plates, smaller glasses, smaller portions
Wait before you eat and go slow
Keep a food diary

Tackle temptation
Use the Proximity Principle
Make healthy foods available
Don't eat from the box
Don't get distracted
Use site-specific aversion therapy
Get a handle on habit
Undermine the status quo with deliberate practice
Make specific commitments, not vague ones
Give yourself positive feedback
Keep the commitment small
Know your triggers
Work on your willpower
    Don't feel bad, feel good
    Say 'I will', not 'I won't'
    Reframe the motivator
    Find a goal role model

Add exercise
Introduce HIT three days a week
Introduce strength training two days a week
Make it happen
Put on your kit in the morning
Keep your trainers by the door
Write a pledge, be specific
Make a list of excuses; make a list of solutions
Monitor your progress
Use your environment
Get up, get out, get going
Stand up and walk around at least once every hour
Have a car-free week
Tell people
Find a friend to exercise with
Get a gadget –
   use the Fast Beach Diet app

If you would prefer to print a larger format version of this planner in A4, or if you would like to give one to a friend, please go to: http://thefastdiet.co.uk/wp-content/uploads/2014/04/FB-PLANNER.pdf

readily overcome by the reward systems in your brain[30]. This 'hedonic eating' may be a response to any number of outside influences: you'll recognise it if you eat for reasons other than hunger. The kicker might be social (shared lunches, communal eating, everyone at the table agreeing to order pudding); it may be environmental (scheduled mealtimes which persuade you that you're hungry simply because 'one o'clock is lunchtime', the arrival of the bread basket at the beginning of a meal), or emotional (comfort eating, the popcorn that makes a movie more of a treat, the tub of ice cream demolished when you're feeling blue). Try, then, to decipher your hunger. Are you really hungry? Or are you overriding your brain's satiety message? Even posing the question can be enough to still the urge

• **Keep the commitment small**. This is the advice of experimental psychologist Dr BJ Fogg at Stanford's brilliantly named 'Persuasive Technology Lab'. According to his research into creating new habits, small steps are more effective than grand gestures: 'The number one mistake people make,' Fogg told the *Huffington Post*[31], 'is not going tiny enough.' If you're trying to make a change in your life, go small. In fact, go minuscule. Make it something that takes almost no effort and nearly no time. 'Just put on your running shoes,' Fogg says. 'That's it. Put them on in the morning every day for five days. You're done.' According to Fogg – and it's an appealing proposition – by breaking down each resolution to discover what the smallest constituent habit could be, your chances of succeeding will be 50% higher than if you leave it woolly and vague

• **Know your triggers**. Recognise – before it happens – when your self-control is likely to dissolve. Discover the cue that drives a poor habit, and change the reward. If you're always ravenous when you get home from work, make sure there's an apple stashed in your bag to eat en route, so that you don't demolish a packet of Digestives as soon as you're through the front door. Have business lunches in the office or in a park, not in a restaurant where they serve the world's best tiramisu. If you're prone to a late-night forage in the fridge, run a bath instead. Know your food fault-lines – it might be chocolate, ice cream, cheese. In my case, it's dough. For six weeks, commit to a moratorium on your nemesis. Don't buy it. Walk past it. Even demonise it. After six weeks without sugar in your coffee, you may find the very idea of it makes you shudder. I certainly can't look a latte in the eye these days – even though I was a devoted fan for years before I discovered 5:2

A word about willpower

What do we really know about willpower? It's a slippery beast, the eel of the mind. But recent studies have provided new insights which make stimulating food for thought, and can offer ways to galvanise you during your Fast Beach Diet.

• In her book *The Willpower Instinct*, Stanford psychologist Kelly McGonigal suggests that self-control shouldn't be seen as a virtue, but as a muscle: it gets tired from use, but regular exercise makes it stronger. This is great news: it means (as we know from experience on the Fast Diet) that the going gets easier if we persevere

• 'Feeling bad' about giving in to a craving only leads to… more giving in. It turns out that self-compassion is a far better strategy than self-flagellation. This has long been our approach on the Fast Diet, but it's worth being explicit about it here: inner acceptance actually seems to improve outer control – while attempts to fight instincts and desires only serve to make them worse. So, recognising that thought suppression really doesn't work, make a positive commitment rather than a negative one: instead of saying No, say Yes; not 'I won't' (eat the muffin), but 'I will' (have the apple)

• Similarly, you can 'reframe the motivator'. Rather than thinking 'Arrgh, I don't want to be fat', focus on 'I'd like to be slimmer, healthier and full of energy'. Consider what you want, frame it positively, write it down and read it every day

• Self-control is, it seems, subject to social control[32]; we are hard-wired to mimic the behaviour of others, even when it comes to a pursuit as seemingly solitary as willpower. Psychologists call this 'goal contagion', and it chimes with our ideas about embarking on the Fast Beach Diet with a friend or a partner, or finding a 'goal role model' (you may well discover one at www.thefastdiet.co.uk). You might, for instance, decide to try a reward technique with a friend – each of you could put £10 in a pot; if one of you gives up, both of you lose. Canny, eh?

And just add exercise…

chapter 5

Adding exercise

It won't surprise you to learn that introducing exercise into the Fast Diet equation is likely to be hugely beneficial. In conjunction with IF, exercise can help you lose weight (fat, in particular), and it will certainly improve your general fitness, strength and health – which, never forget, is the overarching goal.

Which exercise is best?

The one you like best. It's the one you'll do.

Even a small amount of 'integrative exercise' can really work wonders – studies show that several five-minute bouts of general activity throughout a day will promote cardiovascular and respiratory health, lower your risk of diabetes and improve your longevity. For some people, it's enough simply to get up and get moving.

If you're up for a greater challenge, now is the time to introduce a more considered exercise plan. Again, commit for the next six weeks, not necessarily beyond. Variety is one of the keys to compliance, so choose two or three different exercises to keep you engaged. It helps if the exercise is time-efficient and can fit easily into your day (which is one of the reasons High Intensity Training gets our vote, as we'll see below). Remember, though, that 'exercise' needn't be formal – even a regular, brisk walk will do. You just have to *do it*.

Can I exercise on a Fast Day?

Yes! Research has shown that even a far more extreme three-day total fast has no negative effect on the ability to perform short-term, high-intensity workouts or longer-duration, moderate-intensity exercise. In fact – and this is worth noting if you already exercise regularly and are aiming for optimal fitness – fasted training can result in 'better metabolic adaptations'[33] (which means enhanced performance over time).

If you enjoy cardio workouts, training while fasting can help your body tap into its fat stores – but running a long race on empty is not advised. If you are not used to taking exercise, then start slowly and listen to your body. During the first week on the Fast Beach Diet, novices should limit HIT until they see how their body responds. Some people, incidentally, find that working out the day after a Fast Day can be more challenging; in which case, perhaps make these your rest days to allow your body to adapt to the previous day's efforts.

When is the best time to exercise?

As readers of *Fast Exercise* will know, if you are interested in performance, late afternoon or early evening may be a better time to work out. However, sports scientists at Glasgow University found that, while morning exercise may feel harder for some people, it can be a great mood-booster, setting you up mentally for the day. Their research[34] showed that women in an 8.15am aerobics class achieved a 50% boost to their feelings of well-being compared with 20% for those who worked out at 7.15pm.

If fat-burning is the aim, as we've seen above, you may well find that you benefit from doing exercise in a fasted state. One recent study, for example, found that working out before breakfast is beneficial for metabolic performance and weight loss[35]. According to its authors, 'Our current data indicate that exercise training in the fasted state is more effective than exercise in the carbohydrate-fed state.'

There is, however, some evidence to suggest gender differences in response to fasted training[36] (men tend to build muscles so long as they work out before their main meal; women tend to respond better to training after a meal). What's more, fasted endurance training may work better for women than fasted weight training.

The truth is we are all different and the best time to exercise is the time that best suits you. What all the experts agree upon is that exercise at any time is better than none at all.

The two fundamentals for Fast fitness

Exercise means different things to different people: a Zumba class, a tennis match, a morning jog around the park. To maximise results on the Fast Beach Diet, it's helpful to consider two key areas, and introduce an element of each into your weekly plan:

• Cardio work, particularly HIT

• Strength training for muscle tone

High Intensity Training (HIT)

Despite increasing evidence to the contrary, there is a persistent belief in the fitness industry that the more time you spend exercising the better. 'Go steady but go long' has been the received wisdom, with the promise that you will thus enter the fabled 'fat-burning zone'. But, as Dr Stephen Boutcher at the University of New South Wales says, 'Most exercise programmes designed for weight loss have focused on steady-state exercise of around 30 minutes at a moderate intensity on most days of the week. Disappointingly, these kinds of exercise programmes have led to little or no loss'[37].

The latest thinking, developed in several studies[38] and familiar to anyone who has read Michael's *Fast Exercise* book, is that we can get many of the important benefits of exercise from just three minutes of intense activity a week.

Michael's initial interest in HIT came from meeting Jamie Timmons, a professor of systems biology at Loughborough University. According to Professor Timmons, 'The truth about exercise is shocking and intriguing. It's shocking that we've been given such prescriptive guidelines by government, yet have known so little. HIT has blown apart the scientific theories… The work that I and others have done so far suggests that, on average, HIT leads to the same end point as high-volume training. But the key is this: HIT is much easier to do.'

Below, you'll find a précis of Michael's approach to HIT. Try it as part of your Fast Beach Diet and you'll gain its myriad benefits with only a short, sharp investment of time. If conventional cardio work is more to your taste – whether it's a spin class or a game of squash – by all means commit to doing that. Anything that gets you moving will be a bonus. But I would also encourage you to give HIT a go.

Why moderate exercise gets mediocre results

It should be straightforward: do more exercise, burn more calories, lose more weight. The problem is that, when it comes to humans, things are rarely straightforward. Part of the problem is that fat is an incredibly energy-dense substance. A pound of fat contains more energy than a pound of dynamite. This means you have to do a lot of exercise to burn even a small amount of it. Most of us have neither the time nor the inclination to do the quantity of exercise required.

What's more, when we exercise, we tend to engage in 'compensatory eating', which rather spoils the plot. Studies show that we often make up for even moderate exercise by eating more[39]. Sometimes a lot more. In fact, the very thought of exercise may encourage us to start eating[40].

But, if exercise alone is not a great way to lose fat, we

do know that combining exercise with a diet is likely to be more effective than either done alone. Over the last decade, studies have repeatedly shown that a few minutes of intense exercise a day can make a huge difference. Unbelievably, there is evidence that just 40 seconds of intense activity can have a significant effect[41].

As Michael discovered, you really can get many of the same benefits, perhaps more, from doing HIT as you can from slogging away at the more traditional approach.

These benefits include:

• Improved aerobic fitness and endurance

• Reduced body fat

• Increased body strength

The studies show that:

• HIT will get you aerobically fitter faster than standard exercise

• HIT will improve insulin sensitivity faster than standard exercise

• If you want to build muscle tone and lose some fat, HIT will be the most time-efficient way to go about it

How does HIT burn fat?
When you push the intensity of a workout, you build more

metabolically active muscle, and, because muscle is efficient at burning fat, your total calorie expenditure soars. This happens mainly because HIT encourages the muscle cells to produce new mitochondria, the power plants that transfer fat into energy and heat. The mitochondria not only burn fat when you are exercising but go on doing so for some time afterwards as your muscles recover.

The metabolic stress caused by HIT also leads to an increase in the production of 'catecholamines' – hormones such as adrenaline and noradrenaline – which lead to much greater fat burning. There are more catecholamine receptors in abdominal fat than in subcutaneous fat, so when you get a surge of catecholamines following a vigorous burst of HIT, they target abdominal fat, increasing the release of fat from visceral fat stores.

HIT and insulin sensitivity

Professor Timmons tested Michael for a number of health indices before he started his HIT programme, and then, after four weeks, he returned to the lab to be retested. One of the main tests was for insulin sensitivity (Michael, as readers of *The Fast Diet* will know, was particularly interested in this result as his father died from complications linked to diabetes).

At his first testing, Michael's insulin sensitivity result showed he was just within what is regarded as healthy tolerance. Timmons pointed to several studies which showed that doing just three minutes of HIT a week could improve insulin sensitivity by 24%. And this is exactly the amount by which Michael's own index improved. Other studies have shown even greater improvements in insulin sensitivity following an HIT regime. One found a 35% improvement in insulin sensitivity after only two weeks[42].

So why is this relevant on your Fast Beach Diet? Insulin sensitivity is what keeps your blood glucose stable. As we've seen in chapter 4, when you eat, your digestive system releases glucose into your bloodstream; this causes the pancreas to release insulin, a hormone that triggers body tissue to absorb circulating glucose. Reduced insulin sensitivity means that the pancreas has to release more and more insulin to keep blood-sugar levels stable. Abnormally low insulin sensitivity is known as 'insulin resistance', a condition that results in high levels of insulin, glucose and fats circulating in the bloodstream. This is a main risk factor for metabolic syndrome, which increases the risk of coronary artery disease, stroke and Type 2 diabetes.

It is not yet clear precisely how HIT affects insulin sensitivity, but Timmons and some other scientists suggest it could be because HIT uses many more muscles than conventional aerobic training. HIT engages 80% of the muscles of the body, compared to around 30-40% during moderate jogging or cycling. One of the effects of exercise is to break down glycogen, a stored form of glucose, in muscles. Removing stores of glycogen makes way for fresh glucose to be taken up from the bloodstream. So the more muscle tissue engaged in exercise, the more space is available for new glucose deposits. As Michael wrote in *Fast Exercise*, vigorous exercise such as HIT creates 'a much bigger sink for the glucose that follows a meal'.

HIT and appetite suppression

HIT also seems to suppress appetite in ways that low intensity exercise does not. One study[43] showed that young men ate fewer calories after high intensity workouts than they did after a bout of moderate exercise. Even more encouragingly, the men reported eating fewer calories on the day *following* the highest intensity workout than they did after the moderate session or after resting. So one of their most striking findings is that if you do very high intensity exercise, the effects of appetite suppression last far longer, well into the next day.

HIT, your way

The joy of Fast Exercise (and what it has in common with the Fast Diet) is that the exertion is only ever short-lived: it's the perfect work out for the time-starved generation. As we've established, any exercise at all is better than none. But if you want to introduce HIT into your six-week plan, here's how to go about it.

• The exact choice of exercise is yours. You may already have a favourite activity or gym session. Now's the time to turn up the dial

• The aim is to do three sessions a week; the temptation may be to do more. Don't

• Remember, this is about quality not quantity. Effort is more important than the amount of time you spend or the number of repetitions you do. Try any of the following:

Outdoor running

To turn a normal run into an HIT session, you'll have to inject real intensity into your workout, which means including a few sprints, preferably up a hill. Uphill sprinting is one of the most effective forms of HIT, but if you are not especially fit, build up to this gradually.

- Warm up by jogging for 1-2 minutes
- Run flat-out up a hill for 10 seconds
- Recover for 1-2 minutes
- Repeat

Increase to three or four 30-second bouts as you get fitter. After running up a hill, avoid jogging back down; walk down instead.

Indoor running

Running on a treadmill burns about 5% fewer calories than running outdoors, due to the lack of wind resistance and because the motorised belt helps to propel you along. So crank up the gradient to make sure you are working hard enough.

Follow the protocol for running outdoors, with warm-up, 10-second bouts and recovery – building up the incline and sprint time as you get fitter.

Indoor cycling

- Pedal gently for 1-2 minutes with the resistance on a low setting
- Then set the resistance level to your limit and go to

your maximum effort level for 20 seconds
• Pedal gently again for a further 1-2 minutes to allow your heart rate to return to normal
• Repeat

If you are unfit or have never tried HIT before, start with two 10-second sprints and build up to two 20-second sprints over several weeks. Increase resistance by 2% every two weeks. Advance to three or four 20-second bouts as you get fitter.

Stair-running

This is fairly low-impact on the knees and feet, and great for buttock- and leg-toning. You'll need several flights of stairs, so perhaps try this at work.

• Bound up stairs for 30 seconds
• Recover for 1-2 minutes
• Repeat

The whole foot should land on the stair, and don't run downstairs. You can, of course, do this on a step machine.

Cross-training

• Warm up for 1-2 minutes
• Set to the highest incline and resistance and go at maximum effort for 20 seconds
• Recover for 1-2 minutes
• Repeat and build up to three reps and 30-second bouts as your fitness improves

Swimming

Swimming is a superlative all-round work out and will give you a defined waist and strong shoulders, but it's important to vary the strokes. Rather than judge by time, judge by distance. A 25-metre length at full pelt is comparable to sprinting for around 30-40 seconds.

• Warm up at a leisurely pace for a length
• 'Sprint swim' for half a length
• Recover for 1-2 minutes
• Repeat

Again, build up the sprinting distance and reps to three bouts as you get fitter.

FOOD AND FAST EXERCISE

• Don't attempt Fast Exercise immediately after eating: the main risk is not cramping but vomiting
• Don't load up on carbs before doing Fast Exercise. There is a widespread belief that carbs are needed to fuel exercise. Unless you are exercising heavily for over an hour at a time, you have plenty of carbohydrates on board
• Similarly, you don't need to load up on carbs after doing Fast Exercise either. You may feel a bit wobbly but, as we've seen above, the point of doing HIT is to deplete your glycogen reserves (the energy stored in your muscles), making way for fresh

glucose to be deposited in the bloodstream, so the last thing you want to do is immediately replenish them. The average person doing a HIT session three times a week does not require special 'refuelling'

IS HIT SAFE?

Michael suggests that if you are unfit you should ease yourself into HIT. Don't exercise if you feel unwell; your body needs its resources to get better. Anyone who has doubts about their health should have a medical check-up before starting any form of exercise.

Strength training

Of course, getting fit is about more than simply doing cardiovascular exercise, whether you take a traditional approach or try HIT. A beach-fit body requires tone and flexibility too. Weight training while fasting can help your body build more lean muscle (particularly if you are male) and maintain bone density. It will give you a lengthened, strengthened figure – exactly what you want as you head for the beach with only a swimsuit for company. The following simple, familiar exercises are just suggestions; you may well have your own favourites. Since you don't need any specialist equipment – just the resistance of your own body weight –

you can do them anywhere, any time. You could do them now. Include some or all of the following exercises, adapted from fitness expert Peta Bee's programme in *Fast Exercise*, on the days when you're not doing HIT.

Push-ups

Lie face down with the palms of your hands directly beneath your shoulders and the balls of your feet touching the ground. Keep your body straight – your head in line with your back – and raise yourself up using your arms. Lower your torso to the ground until your elbows form a 90-degree angle and then push up again. If you find this too challenging, do it with your knees on the ground until you are strong enough to perform full push-ups.

Jumping jacks or star jumps

You'll remember these from PE lessons at school, and there's something joyful about doing them in the kitchen while you're waiting for the kettle to boil. Stand with your hands by your sides. In one movement, jump up with your legs apart as you raise your arms to the sides. Land with your arms over your head and your feet more than hip-width apart. Jump up again and, in one movement, bring your legs together and your hands back to your sides.

Wall-sit

Start with your back against a wall with your feet shoulder-width apart and positioned about two feet from the wall. Slowly slide your back down the wall until your thighs are parallel to the ground and your knees are directly above your ankles. Don't arch your back. Hold the position for as long as you can

Ab crunches

Lie on your back with your knees bent, your feet flat on the floor and your hands positioned either side of your head. Raise your upper body without lifting the lower back off the ground, making sure your chin is tucked in towards your chest. When your shoulders and upper back are lifted off the floor, gently curl back down.

Squats

Stand with your feet shoulder-width apart and hands placed lightly on opposite shoulders. Imagine you are preparing to sit in a chair; bend at the knee, keeping the weight in your heels. Make sure your back is as straight as possible. Keep bending until your legs make a 90-degree angle, with your thighs parallel to the ground. Push back up without bending your back.

Plank

Lie on your front on the floor and then raise yourself onto your forearms and toes so that your body forms a straight line from head to toe. Make sure your mid-section doesn't lift or drop. Hold the position for as long as possible. Remember, it should never cause pain in your lower back.

Lunges

Stand with your back straight and your feet shoulder-width

apart. Stride forward with one leg, bending both knees to 90 degrees and keeping your upper body straight. Pull back to the starting position and repeat with the other leg.

Do as many repeats of each exercise as you can manage in 30 seconds and take a 10-second rest between each bout. Again, over the six weeks, aim to increase the number of reps, and/or the length of each bout.

FINDING FLEXIBILITY AND STRENGTH THROUGH YOGA AND PILATES

Yoga and Pilates, among their many benefits, will bless you with a stronger, leaner body. They also aid posture, balance and core strength. Dynamic yoga such as Astanga or Bikram will give you a more intense workout, but regular practice of any form will help strengthen and define muscles, particularly if you hold the poses – Down Dog, Plank and Chaturanga Dandasana (a yogic push-up) can be challenging and intense, particularly as a dynamic sequence in the Sun Salutation. Yoga will also put you in touch with your body, something that can get overlooked when we reside mainly in the mind. Noticing (not judging) how your body feels and reacts on any given day, right now, is the basis of good yoga practice and a crucial starting point for the Fast Diet. Including meditation and breathing practice will support your mindfulness mission. As a yoga nut with 20 years of practice behind me, I strongly advise that you find a teacher who speaks your language and inspires you. Pilates, too, will help streamline a body. You'll gain spine mobility and core strength, together with improved skeletal alignment. All good.

Everyday exercise: what to do when on the Fast Beach Diet

Aim to introduce HIT three times a week. You can choose which days suit – as we've seen, there's no reason to avoid exercise on a Fast Day. But find a balance that seems to work for you. Again, apply the motivator that this is just for six weeks: it's a means to an end. You may well find that exercise, in whatever form, soon becomes an integral and enjoyable part of your life.

On two other days, introduce strengthening exercises whenever and wherever you can. Five minutes of push-ups and plank before bed. A half-hour yoga session before you start work. Lunges and crunches in front of your favourite TV soap. Whatever you can do, do. Just ensure that you have two rest days, free of exercise.

How to bring exercise into your life

It's all very well to make a plan. But how to make it happen?

Sometimes, as we discovered when looking at habits in chapter 4, it's enough to shift your perspective by doing small, seemingly inconsequential things...

• **Put on your exercise kit, not jeans, first thing** – and keep your trainers handy. Just as you are more likely to eat crisps if they're in full view, so you are more likely to exercise if the cues are staring you in the face. Put your running shoes by the front door, move the exercise bike into the family room; find somewhere else to hang your washing other than on the cross-trainer. As Dr Fogg's investigations have shown, tiny steps such as these can change the clockwork routine of your day

• **Write a pledge, and make it as specific as you can**. 'I will do a 5-minute session of HIT on the exercise bike, three times a week starting tomorrow evening when I get back from work' would be a good start. Pin it on the wall, schedule it into your diary, put reminders on your phone, tell your kids. Whatever works for you, but the more clearly you have thought it through, the more likely you are to do it

• **Write a list of potential excuses**... Can't find shoes, running clothes in the wash, I'm tired, it's cold, the football's on the telly... Now address each in turn and write down the solutions. Anticipating potential barriers reduces the chance of back-sliding

• **Monitor your progress**. Remember the power of positive feedback? Remember the benefits of keeping a food diary and logging your achievements? The same goes for exercise. Download an app that appeals to you (the Fast Beach Diet app will help you track your work-outs), or use the pull-out planner included in this book

• **Take advantage of your environment**. Use that park bench, tackle that hill. Or you could simply embrace one of Michael's pet projects and *always take the stairs*. Some time ago, I came across a comment from British architect Will Alsop: 'If you really wanted to do something about [the obesity crisis],' he said, 'You could take all the elevators out of all the buildings in London. Then people would be fit'[44]. He's not wrong. When employees of the University Hospital of Geneva were banned from using the lift for 12 weeks – a move that increased their daily climb from five to 23 flights of stairs – their aerobic capacity increased by an average of 8.6% and their body-fat levels fell by 2%[45]

• **Get up, get out, get going**. We apparently spend an average of 14 hours and 28 minutes a day sitting down – the equivalent of 36 years of our adult lives[46]. Allowing for eight hours' sleep, we spend a meagre hour and a half on our feet, active, each day. Researchers have found that, after a day without movement, lipase, an enzyme that helps the body break down fat, is suppressed, almost to the point of shutting off. When we sit, fat is more likely to be stored as adipose tissue than be passed to the muscles where it can be burned. Sitting for prolonged periods thus results in the retention of fat, a lower HDL (that's the 'good cholesterol') and an overall reduction in the metabolic rate[47]

So, try a few tiny tricks to make a stand:

• Go and see a colleague instead of sending an email

• Stand up and pace about while talking on the phone

• Drink plenty of water. This not only keeps you hydrated but it also increases the need for loo breaks, which means in turn more short, brisk walks

• Have a car-free week: a study[48] of 11,000 Atlanta residents reported a correlation between driving and weight gain, with every additional hour spent in a car each day associated with a 6% increase in the likelihood of obesity. For the next six weeks, leave the car at home whenever you can

• Tell people. Publicly stating a goal makes you more likely to follow through, especially, it seems, if you are female

• Exercise with others. If you're planning on going for a jog or a walk, invite someone to do it with you. One of the main reasons people employ personal trainers is to have someone to get them out of the house when they don't feel like going

• Get a gadget. Pedometer use is associated with significant increases in physical activity and decreases in BMI and blood pressure[49]. Fitness apps – you could try the Fast Exercise app – are likely to have a similar effect

THINK YOURSELF FIT

Exercise and its benefits are all in the body, right? But what if they're also in the mind? A fabulous piece of research in this area came from Harvard's psychology department in 2007[50]. It involved 84 female hotel attendants from seven hotels, each of whom cleaned an average of 15 rooms a day. Despite this being hard, physical labour, 66% of the women reported that they did not exercise regularly. More than 36% said they got no exercise at all.

The researchers then divided them into two groups, giving one group detailed information about the calorie burn and health benefits of the activities such as vacuuming and cleaning that they undertook every day. After a month, the tutored group perceived that they did more exercise than before, while the untutored group's responses were unchanged. Neither group had altered their actual level of activity.

But here's the fascinating bit: despite no change in exercise level, the tutored group showed 'improvement on every single one of the objective health measures recorded: weight, body fat, body mass index, waist-to-hip ratio and blood pressure'. They had lost an average of 2lbs and lowered their blood pressure by almost 10%. Just something to think about the next time you pull on your trainers for a session of HIT...

chapter 6

My Fast Beach Diet diary

So, now that you have a real feel for the Fast Beach Diet, it's time to get down to the nitty-gritty. What happens on a day-to-day basis? What can you expect? Here's a typical 'week in the life' of the Fast Beach Diet for me, together with approximate calorie counts (your schedule will, of course, differ, but notice the amendments I've made to take in as much exercise and as many 'good' habits as possible).

Sunday
Non-Fast Day
HIT Day 1

Morning: toast and honey (I have wholemeal bread and stop at one slice rather than my habitual two), peppermint tea, half a mango with lime

Afternoon: Sunday lunch with the family at the pub (I order a child's portion of roast beef and don't have pudding), followed by a proper, long walk with the dog on the Downs; we race each other to the top of the hill

Evening: I'm not particularly hungry in the evening, so I have veggie soup from the freezer, with a slice of wholemeal bread and a bit of goat's cheese. Once the kids are in bed, instead of watching TV, I do a HIT session on the exercise bike. *Then* I watch TV

Total calories: approximately 1,600 – no need to count every calorie, just be gently 'aware'
Total exercise: long walk and HIT

Monday
Fast Day 1

Morning: porridge and berries for breakfast, black coffee; half-an-hour of stretching and strength exercises

Afternoon: no lunch. I'm a bit hungry, so I eat an apple, pips and all. More black coffee, peppermint tea. Busy at work, time flies

Evening: harissa-spiced chicken breast with a huge pile of salad – lots of different leaves and seeds. Early to bed; tomorrow's another day

Total calories: 500
Total exercise: stretching and strength exercises

Tuesday
Non-Fast Day

Morning: scrambled eggs and a wholemeal tortilla for breakfast. I take the dog for a brisk walk along the beach, walking fast enough to be slightly out of breath

Afternoon: out for lunch with friends. I walk rather than drive, just for a change (no parking fee!). I order baked cod with cherry tomatoes and Puy lentils, no bread, no pudding. Fizzy water with fresh lime

Evening: Pilates class 6pm. Family supper of spaghetti bolognaise. I have a small portion, and fill half of my plate with veg – broccoli, sugar snaps and peas. Natural yoghurt with toasted hazelnuts and a swirl of honey

Total calories: around 1700 – again, no need to be particular about counting
Total exercise: walking the dog, walking all day (no car), Pilates class

Wednesday
Non-Fast Day
HIT Day 2
Meat-free day

Morning: porridge with cinnamon and nuts for breakfast, black coffee, water

Afternoon: a busy day at work, so I have lunch at my desk: sashimi and edamame from Yo! Sushi and a sachet of miso soup, plus plenty of sparkling water

Evening: not as hungry as I was expecting. I have cauliflower cheese for supper, but no crispy bacon. I don't have seconds. Half a cantaloupe melon, some blueberries and handful of almonds. A session of HIT – uphill running, 15 minutes – followed by half-an-hour of yoga

Total calories: around 1200
Total exercise: HIT session, half-an-hour of yoga

Thursday
Fast Day 2

Morning: I have an early work meeting – so I arrange to have it on the move down by the seafront, not at a restaurant. No breakfast, but plenty of water and chamomile tea

Afternoon: No lunch

Evening: Tuscan summer bean soup and a small portion of Thai beef salad (see chapter 7). Stretching and strength exercises (star jumps, push ups and plank), half-an-hour of yoga, then early to bed

Total calories: 525

Total exercise: walk along the seafront, take stairs not lifts all day, stretching and strengthening exercises, yoga

Friday
Non-Fast Day

Morning: breakfast on the go as I have to catch an early train – small fruit salad pot and instant porridge from M&S, black coffee from Pret

Afternoon: no time for proper lunch, but grab some oat cakes, an apple and Gruyère cheese; plenty of sparkling water. Don't take the Tube, but walk between meetings. Take the stairs (quickly) at the station. I buy a green juice on the way home

Evening: takeaway curry with the family. I have a chicken tikka with plain rice, not pilau, and tarka dahl (lentils) and okra (ladies' fingers). No naan

Total calories: around 1700
Total exercise: stair climbing and pavement walking

Saturday
Non-Fast Day
HIT Day 3

Morning: quick session of HIT before breakfast to see

what 'fasted training' feels like. Quite hungry afterwards, but make a point of not eating fast-release carbs. Have poached eggs on slice of toast, followed by yoghurt and chopped pear. Black coffee

Afternoon: dog walk on the Downs. Lunch with the kids – we have a tricolore salad – avocado, mozzarella, cherry tomatoes and baby spinach leaves. I leave the bread and pud to the children, but have a small handful of grapes and pistachios with my peppermint tea.

Evening: out with friends – decide not to stay out for dinner (I have grilled salmon with green beans and olives – 'O'Kelly fish' – at home) and go to the movies instead. I drink water, not fizz, and share a small bar of Green & Black's Maya Gold (rather than buying the big size)

Total calories: around 1600
Total exercise: HIT cycle session, dog walking

You'll notice that there's no alcohol and not many snacks on my list. Remember, this plan is only six weeks long. You can do it.

chapter 7

The recipes

Simple summer food... the perfect fit for the Fast Beach Diet

Like many people, I find fasting so much easier in summer. Not only are the fresh seasonal ingredients perfect for Fast Day dishes, the heat (when it comes) also serves to take the edge of an appetite. Most of us don't hunger for carbs and cake when the temperature rises; what we're after are sharp, clean flavours and snappy cooking, the kind that lets us spend more time outdoors and less time glued to the hob.

In summer, plenty of Fast Dieters will eat simple grilled fish or meat – perhaps marinated in chilli and spice, or lemon and herbs – alongside a great mass of salad leaves or steamed greens. Others prefer to embark on something with a bit more pizzazz. The recipes here will broaden your repertoire and give your mouth something to think about on a Fast Day. But first, what's for breakfast?

breakfast

Fast Day muesli
120 calories per 30g portion

Try making your own low-GI muesli with plenty of seeds and nuts. It's satiating and tasty, but quite calorific (blame the nuts), so use sparingly, more as a topping than a base. And stick with it: once you've trained your taste-buds to enjoy this infinitely superior Fast Day version, the shop-bought sugared varieties won't get a look-in.

   100g whole oats
   100g rye flakes
   30g oat bran
   2 tbsp each sunflower seeds, pumpkin seeds,
      linseed, poppy seeds
   2 tbsp each almonds and hazelnuts, roughly
      chopped
   2 tbsp coconut flakes (for sweetness)

Combine the ingredients – this makes about 360g – and keep the muesli in an airtight container (you can, of course, multiply the quantities).

**Fast Day muesli with fresh strawberries
and yoghurt**
245 calories per portion
Serves 1

    30g Fast Day muesli
    100g low-fat natural yoghurt
    10 strawberries

Add a handful of muesli to yoghurt and top with strawberries.

Oat berry smoothie
220 calories per portion
Serves 1

Oats are full of soluble fibre and release energy slowly to set
you up for the day (use jumbo oats rather than the more
finely milled varieties).

    75ml skimmed milk
    100g low-fat Greek yoghurt
    25g jumbo porridge oats (3 tbsp)
    50g blueberries or raspberries

Put all ingredients in a processor and blitz. Alternatively,
leave out the berries (-25 calories) and try the oat base with:

- Chopped dates (+46 calories for two) and apricots (+24 calories for three halves of dried fruit)
- Honey (+22 calories per tsp) and 1 tbsp fresh blackberries (+15)
- Chopped pear (+103 calories per pear) and nutmeg
- Apple (+72 calories per medium apple), cinnamon and vanilla extract
- Banana (+105 calories) and honey (+22 calories per tsp)

Another way to add sweetness is to use low-lactose cow's milk, which is slightly sweeter on the palate than regular milk. Or try almond milk for a non-dairy alternative.

Scrambled eggs
220 calories per portion
Serves 1

   2 medium eggs
   1 tbsp milk (optional)
   ½ tsp butter
   Sea salt and pepper

Beat the eggs with milk, sea salt and freshly ground pepper. Whisk well. Melt butter in a small non-stick pan and cook very gently, stirring all the time. Remove from heat.

Serve with...

• Smoked salmon (+90 calories for 50g) or flakes of hot smoked trout (+70 calories for 50g)
• Turmeric, cumin, finely chopped spring onion, a little green chilli and a chopped ripe tomato (+20 calories)
• Seed mustard (+15 calories per tbsp)
• Pesto (+135 calories per tbsp), a crumble of feta (+69 calories for 25g) and a scatter of fresh basil leaves
• Torn watercress and a dash of balsamic vinegar
• A handful of rocket and sliced pimentos (+12 calories for 50g)
• Parmesan (+60 calories for 15g) and anchovies (+20 calories for 4 drained fillets) – grate the cheese, chop the fish, add to the egg mixture before cooking
• Prawns (+36 calories for 50g) and coriander

Poached eggs

180 calories per portion
Serves 1

2 medium eggs
1 tsp white wine vinegar

Boil a large pan of lightly salted water and keep at a simmer over a gentle heat. Crack a medium egg into a cup. Swirl the simmering water, add vinegar to help the egg white coagulate; then gently add the egg. Poach for 2-3 minutes or until set to your liking. Remove from the pan with a slotted spoon and set it to dry on kitchen paper.

Serve with…

• Parma ham – trimmed of fat (+80 calories for 2 slices)
• Spinach – loosely chopped spinach. Heat 10g butter (+75 calories) in a small frying pan and flash fry for a minute. Perhaps add a pinch of chilli flakes, a finely sliced spring onion and a squeeze of lemon (which will help the vitamins in the spinach to be absorbed)
• Smoked kipper fillets: to cook with no smell, place fish in a microwaveable dish, add a slice of lemon, cover with cling film and microwave for 2½ minutes or until cooked through (+232 calories for 100g)

Boiled eggs
90 calories per egg
Serves 1

Take a medium egg, place in a pan of cold water, bring to the boil and allow to simmer for 3-4 minutes, or until cooked to your liking.
Serve with…

• Asparagus spears – trim 5 asparagus spears and either add to the boiling water with the egg, or steam for 3-4 minutes

---

Tricolore omelette
184 calories per portion (216 with cheese)
Serves 1

Go for goat's cheese if you can, as it has fewer calories and less fat than the average cheese made from cow's milk: 80 calories and 6g of fat per ounce, compared to around 100 calories and 10g of fat per ounce. This is a fine way to get punch and flavour into what could be a bland dish; include the cheese to get the full taste and tricolore effect, but leave it out if calories are scarce.

    2 medium eggs
    1 spring onion, finely chopped
    ½ tsp chilli flakes
    Cooking oil spray
    Salt and pepper
    10g goat's cheese (optional)
    Curly parsley, chopped

Lightly fry the spring onion and chilli flakes (as many or

as few as you fancy) in a small frying pan with just a spray of oil to prevent sticking. Beat the eggs with a fork until bubbly. Add salt and plenty of pepper, and cook gently until the omelette is set to your liking. Add a crumble of goat's cheese and the chopped parsley to serve.

supper

Fish

Deb's monkfish with roasted peppers and tomatoes
289 calories per portion
Serves 2

Monkfish tends to be fairly expensive, but this is one of those dishes with a bit of drama and delight. A Fast Day Special...

    2 monkfish fillets (approx. 200g each)
    4 ripe summer tomatoes – the best you can get
    2 tsp olive oil
    2 tbsp balsamic vinegar
    Sea salt and black pepper
    1 garlic clove, finely chopped
    2 red peppers, left whole
    Handful of fresh basil leaves
    4 slices of Parma ham, fat removed

Preheat the oven to 180°C. Cut tomatoes around their equator and place on a baking tray. Drizzle with the olive oil and balsamic vinegar, season and dot with chopped garlic. Place whole peppers in the pan alongside tomatoes. Roast for 30 minutes until softened and slightly charred. Set tomatoes aside, and place cooked peppers in a bowl. Cover with clingfilm and allow to steam. Once cooled, ease off the skin and deseed, then cut into wide strips.

Clean the monkfish fillets, removing any membrane, and dry well. Gently season them. Place 4-5 strips of roasted pepper on one fillet, and top with 4 or 5 basil leaves. Lay the remaining fillet on top and wrap the parcel firmly in Parma ham, securing with toothpicks if necessary.

Cook in the hot oven for 20-25 minutes or until cooked through (this will depend on size and thickness of the fish; check after 20 minutes). Leave it to rest for 5-10 minutes. Meanwhile, purée remaining peppers in a blender, together with the roasted tomatoes and more fresh basil. Either serve at room temperature, or warm the purée in a small saucepan on a low heat; season to taste. Slice fish into four medallions and serve drizzled with pepper purée. A salad of soft leaves would be nice too.

Italian seafood salad
261 calories per portion
Serves 4

Lightly poached seafood makes an ideal, and incredibly simple, Fast Day supper. Buy it fresh or frozen, cook it quickly and serve at once.

As an alternative, this salad is just as good with an Asian kick – just use chopped coriander instead of parsley and chives, lime juice to replace the lemon, and a mix of sesame oil and olive oil. A scatter of sesame seeds would seal the deal.

400g raw shell-on prawns
400g mussels
400g squid rings

For the dressing
Juice of a lemon
2 tbsp extra virgin olive oil
1 garlic clove, crushed
1 tbsp flat-leaf parsley, roughly chopped
1 tbsp chives, snipped
¼ tsp chilli flakes (or more to taste)
Sea salt and freshly ground pepper

For the salad
1 red onion, very thinly sliced
1 bag of baby herb leaves

Mix the dressing ingredients and set aside. Bring a large saucepan of water to the boil, add seafood – the squid last as it cooks the quickest – and simmer gently for 2 minutes or until just cooked through. Drain and discard any mussels that have not opened during cooking. Remove them from their shells and peel the prawns. Place all the seafood in a bowl and pour dressing over it. Chill for 30 minutes and add to the salad ingredients. Serve with lemon slices.

Clara's prawns on toast

310 calories per portion
Serves 2

I don't usually add unnecessary carbs to a Fast Day recipe, but here, the ciabatta is a worthwhile addition – chiefly because it acts as a raft, soaking up all those tangy flavours. You can, of course, leave it out if you prefer.

300g shelled king prawns, cooked

For the dressing
1 tsp fresh root ginger, grated
2 garlic cloves, finely chopped
1 green chilli, deseeded and finely chopped
  (more or less to taste)
Handful of fresh coriander, chopped
Handful of basil leaves, chopped
Juice of half a lemon
2 tbsp extra virgin olive oil
Sea salt and freshly ground pepper

2 slices of ciabatta, to serve

Combine prawns and dressing ingredients and refrigerate for 30 minutes. Toast ciabatta and top with the prawn mixture. Serve.

If you have calories to spare, half a chopped avocado would be welcome in the mix. Add 120 calories per portion.

Sticky fish with ginger and lime and a courgette salad

335 calories per portion with salmon; 219 calories with white fish
Serves 2

This works well with most fish – but is probably best friends with salmon, which happens to have a higher calorie count than white fish. In terms of sustainability, you can't beat tilapia, but take advice from your fishmonger about what is the best fish to place on this bed of herby, tangy veg.

2 fish fillets (approx. 100g each)

For the sauce
1 red chilli, very finely chopped
1 tsp fresh root ginger, grated
2 tsp runny honey
½ garlic clove, crushed
½ lemongrass stalk, tender heart only, very finely chopped
2 spring onions, finely sliced
2 tsp Thai fish sauce
2 tsp soy sauce
Salt and pepper

For the salad
2 small courgettes, peeled into long ribbons
100g bean sprouts

Handful coriander
Handful mint leaves

Preheat oven to 180°C. Mix sauce ingredients. Season fish fillets, place in a small roasting pan and spoon 2 tsp of the sauce on top of each. Bake for 15 minutes, or until cooked to your liking. Combine salad ingredients with the remaining sauce. Serve alongside the baked fish, drizzled with any further juices from the pan.

Salmon tartare, raw and smoked

282 calories per portion
Serves 1

The combination of raw and smoked here is truly delicious, and rather sophisticated too. Dill, with its delicate green tendrils and mild anise flavour, is an ideal companion; it must be fresh, though. Dried dill is a dead loss.

100g raw salmon fillet, very fresh, chilled and
  finely chopped
2 tsp soy sauce
½ tsp fresh root ginger, grated
50g smoked salmon, finely chopped

For the dressing
2 tsp lemon juice

Grating of lemon zest
2 tbsp low-fat natural yoghurt
Snipped chives and chopped dill leaves
1 tsp capers, rinsed and finely chopped
Dill to garnish

Mix raw chopped salmon fillet with soy and ginger, cover and set aside in fridge to marinate for 10 minutes. Add chopped smoked salmon and return the mixture to the fridge. Mix dressing ingredients. Spoon the dressing over the chilled tartare, and top with a generous scattering of dill.

Meat

Spiced chicken with warm lentils and roasted garlic
399 calories per portion
Serves 4

A hearty, tasty dish that's good to eat with friends on a warm summer evening. Don't be alarmed by the quantity of garlic – it softens and sweetens during cooking and adds an unctuous, squashy quality to proceedings.

For the marinade
3cm fresh root ginger, grated

1 tsp ground coriander
1 tsp ground cumin
1 tsp paprika
1 tsp ground turmeric
Juice of a lemon
2 tsp olive oil
Salt and pepper

1 medium chicken (approx. 1.5kg)
1 head of garlic, sliced in half across the equator
125g Puy lentils, washed
2 tbsp water
Generous handful of parsley, chopped
Generous handful of coriander leaves, chopped
1 tbsp chives, snipped
Juice of half a lemon
Sea salt and freshly ground pepper

Whisk marinade ingredients together and rub into chicken, working under the skin. Refrigerate for an hour, or overnight if possible. Preheat oven to 180°C. Place chicken and garlic in a roasting pan and roast for an hour and 10 minutes – or until the juices run clear. Remove garlic and chicken from oven and allow to rest on a separate plate, retaining the juices in the pan. While the chicken is cooking, place lentils in a saucepan, cover with water and boil; when cooked but still al dente, drain and refresh with cold water, drain again and add them to the roasting pan along with 2 tbsp water. Heat through, scraping the pan for tasty, sticky bits on the base. Remove from heat and add chopped herbs and lemon juice. Stir well, season and serve in a generous mound with the carved or torn chicken (with skin removed) and soft garlic.

Chicken and mango salad

418 calories per portion
Serves 2

A light, bright and totally tasty update on coronation chicken – made in minutes and probably demolished in seconds (though I would advise relishing every forkful).

8 chicken mini fillets (approx. 300g)
Olive oil spray
1 tsp curry powder – mild, medium or hot, to taste

For the dressing
4 tbsp low-fat Greek yoghurt (2% fat)
2 tbsp mango chutney
1 tsp curry powder
Zest and juice of a lime
2 tsp water (if you prefer a runnier dressing)
Salt and pepper

For the salad
2 little gem lettuces

100g sugar snap peas, blanched for 2 minutes in
    boiling water and refreshed in cold
1 ripe mango, peeled and sliced
½ small red onion, very finely sliced
Handful of coriander, roughly chopped
1 green chilli, deseeded and finely chopped

Heat oven to 180°C. Spray the chicken pieces with a little olive oil, season and dust with curry powder. Place in a small foil-lined tray and bake for 10-15 minutes until cooked through. Once slightly cooled, tear or slice into bite-sized pieces. Combine dressing ingredients in a bowl and add the cooked chicken. Assemble the salad ingredients, top with the chicken mixture and a final scatter of fresh coriander.

Lime and herb chicken salad
195 calories per portion
Serves 1

Just about my favourite Fast Day food. This is what it's all about: minimum calories, maximum taste.

1 small chicken breast, skin on
A little olive oil
Salt and pepper
½ small cucumber, cut in half lengthways, deseeded
    and cut on the diagonal into crescents

Handful coriander, including finely chopped stalks
Handful mint leaves
½ tbsp Thai fish sauce
1 tbsp lime juice
1 spring onion, finely sliced on the diagonal
½ tsp Szechuan peppercorns, crushed
½ tsp sesame oil
Iceberg lettuce (80g), torn
Lime wedges

Season chicken and rub it lightly with the oil. Bake until cooked through and juices run clear – about 20 minutes. Leave to rest. Remove the skin, tear chicken into shreds and place in a bowl with cucumber, coriander and mint. Stir in fish sauce, lime juice, spring onion, Szechuan pepper, sesame oil, and seasoning. Toss well. Serve on torn iceberg lettuce and garnish with lime wedges and coriander leaves.

Thai beef salad
351 calories per portion
Serves 2

One we know and love, but an ideal choice for a quick, filling and (most crucially) pleasing Fast Day summer supper. Keep the beef rare and thinly sliced. If you're eating with friends, multiply the quantities and perhaps cook your steak on the barbecue.

350g sirloin steak, cut thick and trimmed of fat (ask
   your butcher),
Juice of half a lime
1 tsp soft brown sugar
Sea salt
Szechuan pepper, ground

For the dressing
2 tbsp lime juice
2 tbsp Thai fish sauce
1 tsp soy sauce
1 garlic clove, crushed
1 lemongrass stem, outer leaves removed, finely
   chopped
1 bird's eye chilli, deseeded and finely sliced (to taste)
2 spring onions, finely sliced on the diagonal
Handful of coriander leaves, roughly chopped
1 tsp soft brown sugar

For the salad
1 cos or romaine lettuce, leaves washed and torn
2 ripe tomatoes, cut into eighths (skins removed if
   you prefer)
½ cucumber, cut in half lengthways, deseeded and
   sliced into crescents
1 medium red onion, finely sliced
Handful of fresh coriander leaves

Heat a griddle pan until it is very hot. Drizzle the lime juice onto the steak, sprinkle with sugar and season with salt and Szechuan pepper. Sear seasoned steak for 2-4 minutes on each side until cooked to your liking*, turning frequently and watching that it doesn't burn (the sugar will caramelise, but will also threaten to char). Rest for 10 minutes. Meanwhile, combine dressing ingredients and assemble salad. Slice steak thinly, place decoratively on salad and serve with plenty of the tangy Thai dressing.

* Guide for cooking steak: for rare meat, sear for 1 minute per 1cm of thickness

---

Veg

Goan aubergine curry
173 calories per portion (250 with brown basmati rice)
Serves 2

  1 tsp cumin seeds, dry roasted in a small frying pan
  2 tsp coriander seeds, dry roasted in a small frying pan
  ½ tsp cayenne pepper
  ½ tsp ground turmeric
  1 green chilli, deseeded and finely sliced
  2 garlic cloves, crushed
  3cm fresh root ginger, peeled and grated

200ml water
300ml half-fat coconut milk
1 tbsp tamarind paste
1 large aubergine, cut lengthways into 5mm-thick slices
Salt and pepper

Crush roasted cumin and coriander seeds in a pestle and mortar. Place in a large saucepan along with the cayenne, turmeric, chilli, garlic, ginger and add the water. Bring to a simmer, then add the coconut milk and tamarind paste. Cook on a low heat for 10 minutes, stirring occasionally, until slightly thickened. Heat grill to medium-high. Place aubergine slices on a foil-lined baking tray and brush with a little of the curried sauce. Grill until they are soft and cooked through, turning once and brushing the other side with the sauce – about 10-15 minutes. Place aubergine in a serving dish, and spoon the rest of the hot curry sauce over. If you want rice with your curry, include 50g brown basmati per person. It's a decent Fast Day source of slow-release carbohydrates, and is nutty and nutrient-rich (+77 calories).

Butternut ratatouille
148 calories per portion
Serves 4

A twist on the classic rat – the butternut brings a new texture and colour to the dish. I'd be inclined to eat it with a spoon.

350g butternut squash, peeled, deseeded and cut into
   3cm chunks
2 tbsp olive oil
1 tsp cumin seeds
Salt and pepper
Cooking oil spray
1 onion, finely chopped
1 aubergine, cut into 2cm cubes
1 tbsp tomato purée
1 400g tin cherry tomatoes
2 garlic cloves, crushed
200g spinach leaves
Fresh basil leaves and 1 tbsp grated
   Parmesan to serve

Preheat oven to 200°C. Place butternut squash pieces in
a small roasting pan with the olive oil. Add cumin seeds,
season well and toss to coat. Bake for 20 minutes until
tender, stirring halfway through cooking time. Spray a
pan with cooking oil, sauté the onion until softened, add
aubergine and cook until lightly browned and cooked
through. Add tomato purée, cherry tomatoes, garlic and
roasted butternut. Season. Stir, cover and cook for 10-15
minutes until thickened and really savoury. Add spinach for
final 2 minutes of cooking time, then serve with a scattering
of torn basil and grated Parmesan.

Red veg

164 calories per portion
Serves 4

2 tbsp olive oil
3 red onions, each cut into 8 wedges
3 garlic cloves, crushed
4 carrots, peeled and cut into 1cm chunks
2 beetroot, peeled and cut into 1cm chunks
300g sweet potato or pumpkin, peeled, deseeded and
    cut into 2cm chunks
1 head of raddichio or red chicory, quartered
Juice of half a lemon
2 sprigs of thyme
1 tsp runny honey
2-3 tbsp water
Handful of fresh basil

In a heavy-bottomed pan, heat the oil, then add the vegetables, lemon juice, thyme, honey and water, and stir well. Cover, bring to a simmer and braise gently until the vegetables start to soften – about 25-30 minutes, stirring occasionally to release any stickiness from the pan base. If it gets too dry, add a further tbsp of water. Season well and serve with torn basil leaves.

Sesame tofu with stir-fry mange tout

345 calories per portion
Serves 1

Tofu needs a punch of flavour to drag it from insipidity:
here, the beloved ginger-chilli-lime trio does the business.

    1 tsp soy sauce
    1 tsp chilli sauce
    100g firm tofu, cut into cubes, dried on kitchen paper
    1 tbsp sesame seeds
    1 tbsp groundnut oil
    1 leek, washed and finely sliced
    2cm fresh root ginger, peeled and julienned
    1 small courgette, julienned
    100g mange touts, blanched for a minute in boiling
      water and refreshed in cold
    Squeeze of lime
    Coriander leaves, to serve

Mix soy and chilli sauce in a bowl and add tofu cubes. Leave
to marinate in the fridge for an hour, then coat them in
sesame seeds. Heat a little oil in a non-stick frying pan and fry
tofu cubes for 2 minutes until golden, turning occasionally
and very gently. Remove tofu from the pan and rest on
kitchen paper. Put the remaining oil in the pan, add the leek
and ginger, with any remaining marinade, and stir-fry until
softened. Add courgette, cook for a further 2 minutes, then
add mange touts. Serve vegetables topped with golden cubes
of tofu, a scattering of coriander and more sesame seeds.

Salads

Watermelon salad with feta and black pepper
214 calories per portion
Serves 4

And now for something completely different... We all know how to throw together a salad, but sometimes unusual ingredients can make a fine marriage. This quick combo uses watermelon – which is full of vitamins and, despite its sweetness, has a low GL thanks to its high water content. With feta and fresh pepper, it's a real summer sensation. Try it and see.

For the dressing
1 tbsp balsamic vinegar
2 tsp Dijon mustard
1 garlic clove, crushed
1 tbsp good olive oil

For the salad
1kg watermelon, cubed
200g low-fat feta cheese, crumbled
1 red onion, thinly sliced
Handful of fresh mint leaves, roughly chopped
Freshly ground black pepper
Sea salt

Combine dressing ingredients. Assemble salad, dress, eat.

Courgette, pea and ricotta salad
181 calories per portion
Serves 4

4 young courgettes, peeled into ribbons
100g just-cooked fresh or frozen peas
100g pea shoots
200g ricotta cheese

For the dressing
Zest and juice of a lemon
2 tbsp extra virgin olive oil
1 tsp runny honey
Salt and pepper

Combine dressing ingredients, assemble salad and dot with teaspoons of ricotta. Drizzle with the dressing and serve.

Carrot, spinach and coconut salad with hot griddle halloumi
254 calories per portion
Serves 2

Olive oil spray
100g reduced-fat halloumi, sliced
Salt and pepper

For the salad
1 bag of baby spinach leaves, roughly chopped
2 carrots, peeled and grated
25g fresh coconut, grated

For the dressing
1 tbsp olive oil
1 tsp black mustard or nigella seeds
Juice of a lime
Juice of an orange
Salt and pepper

Spray halloumi slices with a little olive oil, season and sear in a hot griddle pan for 30 seconds on each side. Serve the dressed salad piled on a plate with the hot halloumi on top.

Pen's beetroot salad
159 calories per portion
Serves 4

My friend Pen swears by the mystic power of her shredded beetroot salad. It may sound a bit low-key, but try it: it's truly a sublime mouthful...

For the salad
3 medium fresh beetroots, scrubbed and roughly grated

3 carrots, peeled and grated
1 small celeriac, peeled and grated
1 green apple, grated

For the dressing
2 tbsp horseradish sauce
2 tbsp olive oil
1 tbsp freshly squeezed lemon or orange juice
1 tsp English mustard
1 garlic clove, crushed
Salt and pepper
1 tbsp sesame or pumpkin seeds, to serve

Dress the grated veggies, top with seeds and serve.

Soups

Tuscan summer bean soup
178 calories per portion
Serves 4

1 tbsp olive oil
1 onion, finely diced
2 celery sticks, finely diced
1 red pepper, deseeded and finely diced

1 carrot, peeled and finely diced
2 garlic cloves, crushed
2 thyme sprigs, leaves picked
2 rosemary sprigs
1 bay leaf
1 tsp smoked paprika
1 400g tin cherry tomatoes
1l good vegetable stock
1 vegetable stock cube
Pinch of caster sugar
1 400g tin cannellini beans, rinsed and drained
1 400g tin flageolet beans, rinsed and drained
100g broad beans, shelled (can be from frozen)
100g petits pois
Salt and pepper

In a large saucepan, heat the oil and add the onion and celery. Sauté until softened, then add the pepper, carrot, garlic, herbs and paprika. Cook, stirring, for a further 3-4 minutes, or until the carrots and peppers begin to soften. Add the tomatoes, stock and stock cube, and a pinch of sugar to bring out the flavour of the tomatoes. Bring to a simmer, then add the tinned beans. Stir gently and simmer for 15-20 minutes; in the final 2 minutes of cooking time, add the broad beans and peas. Bring back to a simmer, season and serve piping hot.

Super-simple fridge gazpacho
113 calories per portion
Serves 2

As fine a summer soup as you could imagine. It matters that the tomatoes are ripe and flavourful. It matters that you eat this fresh from the fridge. After that, nothing else matters at all.

1 red pepper, deseeded and coarsely chopped
300g red tomatoes, ideally a mix of varieties
½ cucumber (150-200g), roughly chopped
1 red chilli, deseeded and roughly chopped
1 garlic clove
2 spring onions, sliced
2 tbsp red wine vinegar
1 tbsp good olive oil
Salt and pepper
Six ice cubes (optional)

Purée all the vegetables together – raw – in a food processor until smooth. Add vinegar, olive oil, ice, salt and pepper and quickly blitz again. Serve cold – with ice cubes floating in it if you wish – with more finely diced cucumber, tomato and spring onion. Gazpacho does not freeze well, so make it on the day and serve fresh.

Vietnamese prawn pho

48 calories per portion (add 10-15 calories for every 50g of additional veg)
Serves 4

Pho is the way to go if you want a big bolt of flavour for very few calories. Add spring vegetables of your choosing – mange touts, sugar snap peas, shredded spring cabbage, ribboned carrots, green beans, shiitake mushrooms or baby sweetcorn… As with all soups, the dish hinges on a good stock.

    2 stems lemongrass, outer leaves removed, finely
        chopped
    2 tsps fresh root ginger, grated
    4 kaffir lime leaves, torn
    1.5l good vegetable stock
    1 tsp palm sugar or light soft brown sugar
    3 tbsp Thai fish sauce
    Juice of a lime
    8 large prawns, shelled and deveined
    50g bean sprouts
    Fresh Thai basil leaves, mint, coriander and finely sliced
        red chilli to serve

Use a pestle and mortar to grind the lemongrass, ginger and kaffir lime leaves. Add the paste to a large saucepan with stock and boil for 10 minutes. Add sugar, fish sauce and lime juice, tasting to check for balance. Cook prawns in broth till they are pink – about 2-3 minutes. Add bean sprouts, plenty of herbs and red chilli to serve. You can also add shirataki noodles at negligible calorie cost: cook according to packet instructions, and ladle the piping hot pho on top.

Don't even think about it…

I included some of these 'Straight to the Plate' ideas in *Fast Cook*, and they proved a popular way to get through supper on a Fast Day with minimum fuss. Not recipes so much as great flavour combinations, these trios can be grabbed from your fridge and kitchen cupboards on days when you just don't want to think too hard about food. Use lemon juice, balsamic vinegar (I like it in spray form) or the basic Fast Day dressing (below) where necessary. Then just add a plate, a fork and an appetite.

• Shredded white cabbage + sliced red onion + hard-boiled egg (1 medium), **100 calories**
• Smoked salmon (50g) + hard-boiled egg (1 medium) + sliced fennel, **180 calories**
• Broad beans (100g) + radicchio + pecorino (30g), **196 calories**
• Lean roast beef (100g) + horseradish crème fraîche (1 tbsp) + little gem lettuce, **203 calories**
• Chicken tikka pieces (130g) + sliced beef tomato + cucumber raita (2 tbsp), **216 calories**
• Avocado (half) + prawns (150g) + low-fat crème fraîche (1 tbsp), **217 calories**

- Parma ham (4 slices) + melon + strawberries, **228 calories**
- Mozzarella (50g) + avocado (half) + 2 ripe tomatoes, **237 calories**
- Baby spinach + Parma ham (4 slices) + Parmesan (30g), **244 calories**
- Low-fat hummus (100g) + raw veggies + jalapeños, **246 calories**
- Tinned tuna (100g) + cannellini beans (100g) + red onion, **268 calories**
- Cooked turkey breast (200g) + rocket + pine nuts (10g), **269 calories**
- Smoked chicken (150g) + romaine lettuce + cashews (20g), **276 calories**
- Blanched French beans + cooked king prawns (150g) + low-fat Feta (100g), **289 calories**
- Roast beetroot (100g) + low-fat halloumi (100g) + rocket, **293 calories**
- Low-fat feta (100g) + hard-boiled egg (1 medium) + red cabbage, **295 calories**
- Pilchards in olive oil (100g) + 10 cherry tomatoes + steamed broccoli florets, **323 calories**
- Smoked mackerel (100g) + watercress + 4 plum tomatoes, **354 calories**
- Beef carpaccio (150g) + toasted pine nuts (10g) + rocket + Parmesan (30g), **404 calories**

The Fast Day dressing
112 calories per tbsp

1 tbsp lemon juice
1 tbsp white wine vinegar
2 tbsp extra virgin olive oil
2 tsp Dijon mustard
1 garlic clove, peeled and left whole
Salt and pepper

Whisk ingredients together and keep in an air-tight jar in the fridge. It will last for a week. Remove garlic clove before eating.

Fast Day snacks

As I have pointed out elsewhere, there's little point in grazing on a Fast Day. But some people need a little lift, particularly in the early days when their appetite is adjusting to the new regime. It's best to avoid easy carbs and go instead for fresh, raw ingredients. Have them prepped and handy in the fridge. Nuts, though high in calories, are full of protein and good fats, and just a few will help you feel full.

- Liquorice root to chew, **0 calories**
- Harley's sugar-free jelly pots, **4 calories**
- 60g cherries, **23 calories**
- 100g blackberries, **25 calories**

- Fresh strawberries, **30 calories for 10**
- A miso soup sachet, or a cup of hot Bovril, **32 calories**
- Crudités: carrots sticks, celery sticks, cucumber sticks, raw pepper, watercress, radishes, cherry tomatoes, approximately **40 calories** per serving
- 1 tbsp cottage cheese, **40 calories**
- Apple slices, including skin and core – add a squeeze of lemon juice, **48 calories**
- 1 tbsp hummus, **56 calories**
- A handful of frozen grapes, **60 calories**
- Pistachios, **60 calories for 10**
- Almonds, **80 calories for 6**
- 60g plain edamame – steamed and served warm with a little rock salt, **84 calories**
- 25g Edam, **85 calories**
- 2 hard-boiled quail's eggs, **90 calories**
- A hardboiled egg, **90 calories** (depending on size)
- 1 tbsp pumpkin and sunflower seeds, **90 calories**
- 25g air-popped popcorn, **148 calories**

FAST DAY COOKING TIPS IN A NUTSHELL

- Feel free to top up the leafy, low-calorie, low-GI vegetables beyond the quantities given in any recipe. It is difficult to pig out on leafy veg, and if you need volume, that's where you should get it
- Some vegetables benefit from cooking, others are best eaten raw. Cooking certain veg – including

carrots, spinach, mushrooms, asparagus, cabbage and peppers – means you are breaking down the cell structure without destroying vitamins, allowing you to absorb more goodness

• Fast Days should be low in fat, rather than no fat. A teaspoon of olive oil can be used in cooking or drizzled over vegetables for flavour, or use a cooking-oil spray to get a thin film. Include a little oil dressing on your salads; it means that you are more likely to absorb their fat-soluble vitamins

• The vitamin C in lemon or orange dressings helps the body to absorb more iron from leafy greens such as spinach and kale. Watercress with orange, for instance, is a great combination

• Cook with a non-stick pan to cut down on calorie-dense fats. Add a splash of water if the food sticks. In summer, bring out the barbecue

• Choose lower-fat cheeses and semi-skimmed or skimmed milk

• Similarly, avoid starchy white carbohydrates (bread, sticky rice, pasta) and opt instead for low-GI carbs such as pulses and slow-burn cereals. Choose brown rice and quinoa

• Ensure that you get plenty of fibre on a Fast Day: eat the skin of apples and pears, have oats for breakfast, keep those leafy vegetables coming in

• Add flavour where you can: chilli flakes will give a kick to any savoury dish. Vinegars, including balsamic, will lend acidity. Add fresh herbs too –

they are virtually calorie-free, but give personality to a plate

• Eating some protein will help keep you fuller longer. Stick to the lean proteins, including vegetable protein from nuts and legumes. Remove the skin and fat from meat before eating

• Use agave as a sweetener if required; it's low-GI

The FBD shopping list: what to have to hand

Get in the habit of having Fast-friendly food around – just enough to allow you to grab a quick meal when you're fasting and famished.

In the fridge

Eggs
Mackerel fillets
Smoked salmon
Half-fat hummus, low-fat natural yoghurt and crème fraîche
Feta, cottage cheese and low-fat mozzarella
Spring onions
Chillies
Fresh herbs
Non-starchy veggies: cauliflower, broccoli, peppers,
    radishes, cherry tomatoes, celery, cucumber, mushrooms,
    lettuce, sugar snaps, mange touts, salad and spinach
Carrots
Lemons
Strawberries, blueberries, apples

In the larder

Tinned tuna, no-drain
Tins of beans and chickpeas
Tins of cherry tomatoes
Tomato purée
Garlic
Onions – red and white
Mustard – Dijon and English
Vinegar – balsamic and white wine; try balsamic spritzer
    on salad
Olive oil
Cooking oil spray
Spices, including cumin and coriander
Chilli flakes
Nuts – unsalted are preferable
Pickles – guindillas, jalapeños, cornichons, capers
Marmite, Oxo cubes, stock cubes, miso paste
Sea salt and freshly ground black pepper
No-sugar Alpen
No-sugar jelly
Shirataki noodles
Miso soup sachets

In the freezer

Root ginger – it is best grated from frozen
Stock, in empty (clean) soup and milk cartons
Soup – home-made or shop bought, in single portions
Blueberries, a cool little snack (strawberries don't
    freeze well)

Six-week meal plan, under 500 calories – breakfast and supper

(for the recipes, see pages 103-137)

WEEK 1	BREAKFAST 100-250 calories	SUPPER 200-350 calories
FAST DAY 1	Poached eggs 180 cals	Goan aubergine curry and brown basmati 250 cals
FAST DAY 2	Muesli, yoghurt and fruit 245	Lime and herb chicken salad 195

WEEK 2	BREAKFAST	SUPPER
FAST DAY 1	Oat berry smoothie 220	Italian seafood salad 261
FAST DAY 2	2 boiled eggs, asparagus 180	Gazpacho 113 and courgette, pea and ricotta salad 181

WEEK 3	BREAKFAST	SUPPER
FAST DAY 1	Scrambled eggs 220	Goan aubergine curry 173
FAST DAY 2	Date and apricot smoothie 280	Lime and herb chicken salad 195

WEEK 4	BREAKFAST 150-250 calories	SUPPER 300-350 calories
FAST DAY 1	Kippers and mushrooms* 234 cals	Watermelon and feta salad 214 cals
FAST DAY 2	Poached egg and ham 170	Sticky salmon with ginger 335

WEEK 5	BREAKFAST	SUPPER
FAST DAY 1	Scrambled eggs, prawns and coriander 356	Carrot, spinach and coconut salad with halloumi 254
FAST DAY 2	Yoghurt, berries, almonds* 264	Tuscan bean soup 178

WEEK 6	BREAKFAST	SUPPER
FAST DAY 1	Tricolore omelette 184	Chicken and mango salad 418
FAST DAY 2	Oat smoothie with apple, cinnamon and vanilla 282	Butternut ratatouille 148

* See *The Fast Diet Recipe Book*

Six week meal plan, under 600 calories – supper only

WEEK 1	SUPPER
FAST DAY 1	Spiced chicken with lentils and garlic 399 calories, served with green salad and Fast Day dressing
FAST DAY 2	Goan aubergine curry and brown basmati 250, served with a shop-bought wholemeal naan 180

WEEK 2	
FAST DAY 1	Pho 48, followed by Thai beef salad 351
FAST DAY 2	Tuscan bean soup 178, followed by sticky salmon with ginger 335

WEEK 3	
FAST DAY 1	Butternut ratatouille 148 with grilled chicken breast 127, green salad and Fast Day dressing
FAST DAY 2	Gazpacho 113, followed by sesame tofu and mange tout stir-fry 345

WEEK 4	SUPPER
FAST DAY 1	Deb's monkfish with roasted peppers/tomatoes 289, served with brown basmati 77 and green beans 20-30
FAST DAY 2	Miso soup 32, followed by sirloin steak 183 with red veg 164 and tenderstem broccoli 40

WEEK 5	
FAST DAY 1	Chicken and mango salad 418
FAST DAY 2	Tricolore omelette 184, followed by Italian seafood salad 261

WEEK 6	
FAST DAY 1	Salmon tartare 282 with courgette, pea and ricotta salad 181
FAST DAY 2	Prawns on toast 310, followed by lime and herb chicken salad 195

chapter 8

Sticking with it in the weeks ahead

So, you've absorbed the new boot-camp method for the Fast Beach Diet. You're energised and raring to go. But what happens in week three and a bit, when you might need a boost? That's the time to turn to friends, and to take yourself to one side for a stern talking-to. Here are practical ways to help yourself out of the rough and into the sunlit uplands of Intermittent Fasting…

Buddy up

A supportive friend may well be one of your greatest assets in the weeks ahead; you might find that they join in, and you'll develop a network of common experience.

Since the plan appeals to men and women equally, couples report that they find it more manageable to do it together (as the testimonials in chapter 9 demonstrate); not only are there anecdotes and experiences to share, but meal times are made infinitely easier if you're eating with someone who understands the rudiments of the plot. It's remarkable how reassuring it is to know that you're not alone.

Go to the forum

What's particularly interesting to me is that the Fast Diet has developed into such a lively conversation. Neither Michael nor I are interested in promoting diet dependency, only in investigating an idea that seems to have truly life-changing potential. Over the past year, that conversation has been evolving and growing online. To tune into the discussion, and to discover countless tips and takes to make the Fast Diet work for you, go to www.thefastdiet.co.uk. Or check out the many Facebook groups – ours is at www.facebook.com/thefastdiet.co.uk

Fast thinking: some final words to get your brain on board

Hold yourself in high esteem

At the risk of sounding like a fridge magnet, here are some of my favourite words from the Buddha which may help to ground and inspire you in the weeks ahead: 'You can search throughout the entire universe for someone who is more deserving of your love and affection than you are yourself, and that person is not to be found anywhere. You yourself, as much as anybody in the entire universe, deserve your love and affection.'

'Do or do not. There is no try'

These words, from Yoda (another favourite), are infinitely wise and work just as well when tackling weight loss as they do in the swamps of Dagobah when contemplating a broken X-wing fighter. The point is to get on with it. No excuses. No attempts. But action. Now. As someone somewhere once said: Just Do It. Go into the next six weeks with your head, and your aspirations, high. But remain playful. So you miss a meal? So what? Just keep going.

Don't give up, you're already part-way there

Having a period in your day when food simply isn't allowed to pass your lips achieves many things, both physiological and psychological. It is galvanising. It can be liberating. It certainly prevents random snacking, and it might also alert you to how often you do this in the normal run of events. Use your success on a Fast Day to inform your actions on a non-Fast Day. Simply realising that you can curb your appetite and cope with a jab of hunger is a great start. You are already on the right road.

Customise

The key – whether you're doing the Fast Diet or the souped-up Fast Beach Diet – is to find a plan that works for you, which means you may need to experiment a little until you find your best fit. Once you've completed the six-week regime presented here, your aim is to arrive at a sustainable, lifelong plan. So relax a little and return to the classic 5:2 Fast Diet. In fact, rather than think of 5:2 as 'a diet', which in its modern usage is larded with quick-fix connotations, perhaps begin to see it as stemming from the classical Greek '*diaita*'. This roughly translates as 'a manner of living'. A way of life. A commitment to health and well-being. As I hope you'll have gathered, there are no promises here, just proposals. Think of them as proposals for a longer, stronger life.

Be sensible, and if it feels wrong, stop

It's vital that this strategy – both the original format and the turbo version – should be practised in a way that's flexible and forgiving. Take each day as it comes. It's OK to break the rules if you need to. If you're concerned about any aspect of IF, see your doctor.

Be kind to yourself

Try not to associate fasting with discomfort; be gentle to cultivate the changes you desire and deserve; don't dwell on the downside, for instance, if a Fast Day is broken. It's no biggie. Move along. Do, however, congratulate yourself, reinforcing the positive feedback loop which, as we saw in chapter 4, really helps when you're trying to break and make habits. Every completed Fast Day means potential weight loss and quantifiable health gain. You're already winning.

As my other guru and fellow Brightonian, Fat Boy Slim, famously sang:

We've come a long, long way together,
Through the hard times and the good,
I have to celebrate you, baby,
I have to praise you like I should.

Dead right. Make this your Shower Song for the next six weeks.

Reward yourself...
With shoes not booze; put the money you save towards... well, how about a new swimsuit? But which one? First, a few friendly tips for women dieters out there...

One piece, madam, or two?

Getting near-naked in front of strangers (or – worse – friends) is one of the great hurdles in a woman's fashion life, whatever her age. So what to wear on that beach once you've completed your Fast Beach Diet and it's time for the great reveal? As a fashion editor, I spent a chunk of my career deliberating on such things in newspapers and magazines, and *The Fast Beach Diet* seems the obvious place to share a few of my favourite beachside tricks.

While a swimsuit gives a sinuous, continuous line, it can also look a bit mumsy, as if you're en route to the public swimming baths with a rubber cap, goggles and a verruca sock. Dare to fling on a bikini (even if you haven't done so in years), and, I promise, you feel immediately racy – off to Amalfi or St Tropez, the wind in your hair and the world at your sandy feet. Get it right and there are three things to love about a bikini: va, va and voom.

According to fashion lore, a bikini is not a bikini unless it can be pulled through a wedding ring – which means that in its meagre embrace, there's nowhere much to hide. A truly great bikini (and you might only ever meet one in a lifetime) can, however, perform untold magic. Here's how to track yours down…

Size

Sounds basic, but do ensure that your bikini is the right size. Always try before you buy; that's what the sticky plastic gusset is there for.

Shape

If you want your bikini to work, rather than simply loaf about on a lounger, look for the following:

• Under-wiring, which will stop your chest heading south

• A top with clip fastenings, not ties: these will give you added stability and enhance your shape

• A tie-side bottom, though, is adjustable and therefore more forgiving than the set-side bikini pants which tend to bite into your behind like a hungry shark

• High-leg bikini bottoms will elongate a leg, but can be demanding; try before you buy, so you arrive at a cut which suits your butt

• As a 46-year-old mother-of-two, I prefer a bikini bottom that has a slightly higher waistband; that extra half-inch of fabric serves to contain a bit of a tummy

• But, counter-intuitive as it may seem, your bottom will appear smaller if you house it in a little less fabric. I'm not suggesting that you go for the Brazilian floss, just something that doesn't completely cover every scrap of flesh as if you've had your arse wallpapered

• A big bust will benefit from a halter top – chiefly because it offers maximum support; you get a great cleavage as an added bonus

• By contrast, bandeaus only really work on flatter chests; on more ample busts, you'll get a curious eruptive effect, like brioche on the rise

Colour

Fashion editors know as a matter of lore that particular colours complement certain skin tones.

• Red is very demanding on almost everyone – leave it to *Baywatch*

• Acid yellow is tricky for pale skin

• The aquas are brilliant for most complexions, with the plus that you'll complement the sea

• Neons are cool, but suit a darker skin tone best. They're also very grabby on the eye, so you'll need buckets of body confidence to pull them off

• White is infinitely more challenging than black. Always

• Chocolate brown is perennially chic; khaki is kind; navy is no-nonsense and benevolent, like a Norton nanny, and a softer alternative to black

• I like a subtle animal-print – something faded in the taupe/stone/biscuit colour range, not the kind of aggressive print that looks as if it's on the attack

• Polka-dots are fun in the sun, but can be infantilising, so wear with caution, or plenty of chutzpah

THE TANNING TRICK

A little lick of sun exposure is no bad thing (it is thought to combat depression and aid sleep); what's more, by some fabulous trick of the light, a tan will lend tone and shave off pounds. Just don't overdo it. Use the correct UVA and UVB protection, avoid sun-beds, and, if in doubt, use a self-tanning product – exfoliating first to avoid those tell-tale Tigger stripes.

TRY THIS FOR THIGHS: A WORD ON CELLULITE

So many products, so little use... I'm not sure that lasers, vacuum massage, micro-encapsulated caffeine tights, infra-red light, retinol serum infusions or radio-frequency treatments will do anything much to help banish the orange peel. So, what might? All of the following are recommended as ways to help combat cellulite. The good news? On the Fast Beach Diet, you'll be doing most of them already...

• Eat more plants and wholegrains
• Cut out processed food
• Drink plenty of water
• Cut back on salt
• Take regular exercise
• Get your circulation going: perhaps try body-brushing and lymphatic drainage massage; the jury's out on how effective they are as anti-cellulite treatments. But they can't hurt, and can feel great

And, last but by no means least...

Some handy advice for men. Your choice of swimwear depends largely on how much you want to reveal and how much you choose to conceal as you stroll from turf to surf.

Speedos
If you are an exceptionally good swimmer, or built like Tom Daley, then Speedos are clearly your beachtime buddy. They are, however, quite unforgiving, leaving very little to the imagination (Stella McCartney joked that Daley's minuscule

trunks were the hardest part of the Team GB's Olympics kit to design because there was no room for the pattern). In their favour, briefs let you swim with ease, dry almost immediately and ensure that you don't take your keys, wallet and phone swimming by mistake. They're also increasingly popular; if you're into manscaping and not averse to a pose, then do feel free.

A bold swirling pattern can easily go a bit Rod Stewart – so look for block colour, with a comfortable mesh inner lining. If, once you've given them a whirl (and, as with all swimwear, do try before you buy), you look less like David Gandy and more Ray Winstone in *Sexy Beast*, perhaps plump for a little more cover.

Trunks

The fitted 'boxer trunk' has been a beachside hit since 2006, when Daniel Craig emerged from the sea in *Casino Royale* wearing his baby-blue Grigioperla mini-shorts. Sales in smaller shorts have been on the rise ever since: according to the bodywear buyer at Selfridges, 'everyone's moving down a shape – boxer-short wearers are moving into trunks, and trunks to briefs. Young, body-conscious men are getting the confidence to wear smaller shapes'. If you're in the market for trunks, look for a retro sports style – Orlebar Brown leads the market here (think Jude Law in *The Talented Mr Ripley*); navy is the best-selling colour at M&S – chiefly because it is unerringly chic without being unduly attention-seeking.

Board shorts

Popular as they may be, board shorts are hardly the most

practical option – the beach equivalent of wearing jeans at the gym. But boardies are cool, and refreshingly modest. If you can cope with the drag through the water, and don't mind surf-dude graphics and a tan line that stops at your knees, they're hot. Try Vilebrequin for that suave Côte d'Azur feel. If you can actually stand up on a surfboard, then look for Aussie brands such as Ripcurl and Billabong, which have got the technical details (stretch fabric, seam reduction, ergonomic cut, quick-dry material, Velcro pockets) just right.

chapter 9

Fast talk: encouragement from Fast Diet fans

Tanya, 41, Berkshire
73lb lost in a year

'At my heaviest, I weighed 17st 6lb! I was so big; I couldn't see how I could ever return to a healthy weight. I'd tried other diets and hated the feelings of guilt when I ate something "naughty". I used to give up and eat more. It was a vicious circle.

'Then, I heard about the 5:2 diet and on January 7th 2013 I started Intermittent Fasting. Initially I did a combination of 5:2 and some weeks 4:3. As the weight came off, the better I felt about myself and the more energy I had. I started walking with a friend on the days I was fasting. This kept me motivated; I used to visualise the differences to my appearance and also the health changes taking place within my body. I've heard that to break a habit (in my case eating) you need to replace it with another habit; mine became fasting.

'I now weigh around 12 stone. That's another thing that's changed; I'm less obsessed with the scales and more interested in how I feel and how my clothes look on my changed body. I have taken the control back over what I eat and when. I understand my body more, know that I have made a massive difference to my health and feel absolutely fantastic!'

Louise Davey, 47, Australia
13lb lost in 10 months
'I have lost six kilos doing 5:2 since April last year. I heard an interview on the radio, downloaded the documentary, went and bought the book. The rest is history. Thanks, Michael. I will be doing this for life now. At first it was to lose some weight, but having watched the documentary online, my main reason for doing the Intermittent Fasting is mental/brain health. Coming from a family with Alzheimer's, I do not want to go down that road. This is good motivation in and of itself, but I do love a challenge. So, making interesting meals and working out how to get through a day is also quite fun. Along the way I have also found many others who do it and have convinced a lot of my friends that this is the way forward if you want to live a long and HEALTHY life.'

Jeanne White, 42, San Francisco, USA
10lb lost in 8 months
'Like many Fast Dieters before me, I'm sure, I fell into this diet, or rather, way of life, after reaching a point that nothing else I was doing was really making a difference. At 42, with two school-age boys, a husband, a home and a full-time job, I felt like I was always on the go and didn't give much thought to calories. As a decades-long non-meat eater, I felt I was "healthy", but gave little thought to the popcorn, chips

or goldfish crackers I'd snack on with my kids after school/
work. After reading about the Fast Diet and watching the
subsequent interviews with Dr Mosley, I thought I would
give it a try. The first two days I chose, a Monday and a
Wednesday, were difficult, I have to be honest! I recall being
in the basement at work and looking at a stack of paper
thinking, "I'm just going to have to eat the paper." But, I
stuck through it, read everything I could find on the Fast
Diet, joined the Facebook page, etc., and came up with a
meal plan that started working immediately.

'I've lost a total of about 10lb since June 2013, and I've
continued with the programme to maintain this healthy
weight. Better yet, I feel great too, full of energy, able to last
through rigorous yoga classes, and sleeping like a baby. I am
an absolute creature of habit, and am quite content eating
relatively similar things daily, so the Fast Diet is easy for me
to stick with, as I've found items that are easy to cook and
that I genuinely enjoy.'

Glory Puljak, 39, Australia
Over 3 stone lost in 8 months
'It's been 8 months now and I've lost 20kg! It just keeps
falling off! This has never happened to me before. I have
never been able to shift this much weight! I love it so much
because I can still have my Friday night drinks and some
dessert on the weekend and my social life doesn't suffer
because of it. I feel so healthy, have so much energy and
I feel so switched on. This, for me, is a life change that I
will continue to do for ever! I cannot thank the Fast Diet
enough! I also need to add that I walk or jog every day! This

just helps me clear my mind and get my heart pumping.'

Joan Rijkels, 67, The Hague, Netherlands
Over 2 stone lost in 18 months

'In January 2012, I went to the doctor for a check-up and was told that I had an 18% chance of contracting a heart or vascular disease; at 20% they prescribe medication to lower cholesterol. My cholesterol level was 6.5 and I weighed 89kg. At 66 years old I decided to make a change to lead a healthier life.

'In August of 2012, I saw Michael Mosley's documentary on Intermittent Fasting. I started immediately. In January of 2013, I bought the book.

'Now it is January 2014, and I weigh 69.7kg. My cholesterol levels have dropped from 6.5 to 3.5 in two years. Also, I have arthritis and my BSE levels (blood sedimentation rate for erythrocytes) which never dropped below 6 for years, dropped to 2 after just six months on the diet.

'This diet has brought benefits to many people in my family: my sister's cholesterol hasn't been this low in 10 years. My other sister and her husband are both on the 5:2 for health benefits as opposed to weight loss, but she has lost 8-10kg, whilst her husband's cholesterol has dropped dramatically. My son-in-law had a triple bypass when he was 30 because of cholesterol problems and within five months of this diet has lost 15kg! My daughter has lost 10kg as well... the list goes on!

'Fasting feels great and I tell everyone that the reason it's sustainable is that if you don't manage to stick to 500 calories on one day... there's always tomorrow!'

Sandi Mueller, 70, Colorado, USA
19lb lost in 10 weeks
'Your diet is the most amazing programme I have ever been on. After 10 weeks, I have lost 19lbs. More importantly, I feel terrific! I have had sinus problems and chronic bronchitis all my life. Now, my sinuses are clear and I can breathe freely. I am 70 years old and I have not felt this vibrant in decades. My 73-year-old husband has lost 20.8lbs and I am certain that his cholesterol level has dropped. His cardiac specialist will be astounded. My sister, who told me about your diet, was able to reduce her pre-diabetic glucose level from 100 to 86 in five weeks. Our youngest daughter with IBS has been symptom-free since her second week on your diet.

'Thank you for taking the time and effort to discover this revolutionary programme. I call it the Fountain of Youth Diet. We all plan to continue this diet for the rest of our lives. You have brought health and hope to millions of people worldwide who could only look forward to a bleak future before your remarkable discovery.'

Ruth Ellis, 45, Yorkshire
3 stone lost in a year
'I chose the Fast Diet for its potential long-term benefits. The fact that it also helps you lose weight was an added bonus. In 12 months I have lost 8 inches off my waist and more than 3 stone in weight. My husband is doing the diet along with me and he has lost over 4 stone.

'On Fast Days, stir-fries and Asian-style soups are our favoured choice, with plenty of vegetables and some protein (chicken, lean meat, prawns, squid, fish). Using spices, herbs and garlic helps to boost the flavour and keep it interesting. I prefer to save most of my calories for the evening meal as I find that if I have something to eat earlier in the day it makes it harder to fight the cravings. I also sleep better if I've had a decent evening meal. If you find yourself feeling light-headed during a Fast Day it's often due to your sodium levels dropping, so a small pinch of salt often sorts that out. The morning after a fast I find it best to have either a protein-based or wholegrain breakfast and not overload on the carbs. When I first started eating this way, I would often overcompensate and eat too much on the non-Fast Days, but over time this settled down and it has helped me to regulate my appetite on other days. I don't worry about calories on non-Fast Days, but I make wiser choices, rarely snack, don't overload my plate and no longer have such a sweet tooth.'

Susie White, late-fifties, Northumberland
Lost 2 inches around waist in 18 months
'At a yearly Well Woman check-up I was told my waist measurement put me just in the "red" and that I should eat less and exercise more. The health warnings were there. I felt pretty down because I eat healthily anyway, garden almost every day and walk quite a lot. For a post-menopausal woman, it is very easy to feel depressed about putting on weight, especially round the middle. I felt it was a gradual process and that it was becoming very hard to reverse.

'The *Horizon* programme came at just the right time; I was impressed by Michael Mosley's scientific approach, and decided the very next week to go for it. It's not so much the thought of living longer but the thought of living fitter and hopefully being a bit less likely to get diabetes or dementia.

'Initial weight loss made me feel so uplifted. There was an immediate feeling of having more energy and my brain feeling sharper. I've followed the Fast Diet ever since, twice a week, except for one day a week over Christmas and New Year. I didn't have loads to lose and I'm very happy with losing a stone. It's the reverse of the depressing downward spiral of putting on weight. Feeling fitter and leaner gives me the spirit to go on fasting. I'm not exaggerating if I describe the Fast Diet as changing my life.'

Kyra Challen, 25, Bedfordshire
12lb lost in first 12 weeks

'When I decided I wanted to try the Fast Diet, one of my main worries was that I would be sitting down to a simple supper and my husband Chris would be there tucking into pizza and chips, so I was surprised and relieved when he suggested we both follow the Fast Diet together. This makes meals easier as we have the same thing, just like on non-Fast Days, and is also really good for my motivation and for sharing ideas about what works and what doesn't.

We still manage our Fast Days differently during the day – he prefers to have breakfast and fast all day, whereas I prefer to fast from getting up until teatime, but come dinnertime we eat together. It is really helpful to know we are both going through the same temptations during the day and it definitely makes me think twice before 'cheating' on a Fast Day.

'Since starting the Fast Diet, the main changes I have

noticed are not just around weight loss: I have more energy and my appetite every day, even non-Fast Days, has dramatically decreased; I just don't want to eat as much any more, which is going to be a life-saving habit, I think. By Christmas I had lost 12lb after following the diet for about 12 weeks and my husband lost 1st 2lb in that same time, so our combined weight loss is about 2 stone. We both fit easily into clothes from a few years ago now!'

Carol Massey

'This diet enabled me in the first week to join in and socialise and still lose weight. I now want to lose my excess weight with three fasts per week. I don't feel daunted by this at all, that is a first. I am so enjoying planning my meals ahead of time. I love a stir-fry and the Fast Days energise me the next day. I am eating healthy food on non-Fast Days and don't feel tempted to overeat.

'It's true what the book says: "my appetite has been retuned". I see how I was eating when I didn't need food but was thirsty. I drink very weak Earl Grey tea all day and never feel hungry, except when it's time for my main meal. I grazed before and see why the weight kept coming back. I now just eat at mealtimes and take time to savour food. And knowing if I really do want a piece of cake I can have it is great. Funnily, the urge for these foods has gone. I made a batch of ginger biscuits the other day and had a couple, then gave the rest away to a grateful skinny friend! Because I know I have a "choice" it changes everything. How great is that?'

Jeff Chinnock, mid-forties, Devon
2 stone lost in a year

'We have been doing the 5:2 diet since September 2012 after seeing the *Horizon* programme. We have stuck to it ever since – apart from a brief Christmas break – and it has completely transformed how we eat, our relationship with food as well as having a positive impact on our health and waistlines.

'My wife has recently been diagnosed with an endocrine disease that usually causes uncontrollable weight gain (and a risk of diabetes) and everyone has said that there is little you can do about this. But by doing the Fast Diet she has managed to maintain and even lose some weight without affecting her nutrition, and she has avoided diabetes.

At the same time, the book has helped to remind me of the original inspiration for adopting this way of eating (not sure I would describe it as a diet) and the tips and recipes have been extremely useful in helping us provide a bit more variety to what we eat. I have lost over 2 stone and feel much healthier – the only downside being the need to buy new clothes...'

From the www.thefastdiet.co.uk forum:

Angie090465
'At first I worried like everyone else about fasting, would I get so hungry I would faint? Would I even last the day?

The only way to find out was to actually go ahead and give this fasting way of life a try! I picked 2 days and I was pleasantly surprised to find that it wasn't as difficult as I had

feared, and the more fasts I completed the easier it became...
I did not loose weight straightaway, this is a common
question from newbies, because when the lbs don't fall off
right away they assume it does not work! But you have to
give it time, at least a few weeks... Istarted losing a few lbs
each month which I was happy about. I started at 9st 13 and
wanted to lose at least 10lbs and I didn't mind how long it
would take as for me this would become a way of life.

'Now it's April 2014 and I am hovering around 9st 5 or
6; I am happy with that and have now switched to 6:1, ie
where you do one fast a week to maintain.

'I do hope my story inspires others to give 5:2 a go, i now
enjoy the health benefits of it, my skin is so much clearer,
I have much more energy and i can get up at 6 am in the
morning without the lethargic feeling anymore!

sylvestra

'I could say I've "only" lost 1lb this week... BUT I started
doing 5:2 to "kick start" my weight loss again after reaching
a plateau. I've been doing 5:2 for three weeks and have lost
FIVE lb in that time – added to my other weight loss, since
February I have lost 40lb in total – that's 20% of my original
weight and I'm two-thirds of the way to my target weight.
It may not continue like this every week but as long as the
trend is downwards I'll be a happy bunny. The 5:2 certainly
does make you rethink your eating. As I posted on another
thread – I started using 'cauliflower rice' and 'courgette
spaghetti' on fast days as they're low on calories, low on
carbs and lighter on the digestion and now find I prefer this
to the real thing which I'm finding stodgy!'

From Twitter:

@follielincoln
Started @TheFastDietBook 1yr ago & lost a stubborn 23lb. Wish the 20 yr old 5-stone heavier me knew what this 40-something does!

@TheFastDietBook
RT from double Olympian @NathanJDouglas 'the #fastdiet is the diet that I recommend to people when they ask my advice, it's a great diet'

@Mrs_Metters
#FastDiet 4 months, 32 fast days, 48000kcal not consumed, 17lb lost, 3 BMI points dropped, #SkinnyJeansOn

@JennieJHill
I've been doing this 4 weeks, have lost 4 kilos, and my bloke has lost 5. Also healthier. It's wonderful

@LucyKStirk
Thanks for your inspiration. Started in Sept and just passed the 3st lost mark! #doesnotfeellikeadiet

@Caffy49
I call it my Guiltless Diet, on my 5 days of normal eating I don't beat myself up if I have an indulgent day. Easy dieting

ENDNOTES

1 Beneficial Metabolic Effects of Regular Meal Frequency on Dietary Thermogenesis, Insulin Sensitivity, and Fasting Lipid Profiles in Healthy Obese Women, by HR Farshchi, Nottingham University, *American Journal of Clinical Nutrition*, January 2005

2 Short-term Modified Alternate-Day Fasting: a novel dietary strategy for weight loss and cardio-protection in obese adults, by KA Varady, S Bhutan, EC Church and M Kempe, *American Journal of Clinical Nutrition*, November 2009

3 Our Liver Vacation: is a dry January really worth it?, by A Coghan, *New Scientist*, 13 January 2014

4 Sainsbury's survey, reported in the *Guardian*, 20 February 2014 http://www.theguardian.com/business/2014/feb/20/sainsburys-wine-label-calorie-counts

5 Shape of Glass and Amount of Alcohol Poured: comparative study of effect of practice and concentration, by B Wansink and K van Ittersum, *British Medical Journal*, December 2005

6 An Insulin Index of Foods: the insulin demand generated by 1000-kj portions of common foods, by SHA Holt, JC Brand Miller and P Petocz, *American Journal of Clinical Nutrition*, 1997

7 Can Low-Fat Nutrition Labels Lead to Obesity?, B Wansink and P Chandon, *Journal of Marketing Research*, November 2006

8 Reward Mechanisms in Obesity: new insights and future directions, by PJ Kenny, *Neuron* 69, 2011
Dopamine D2 Receptors in Addiction-like Reward Dysfunction and Compulsive Eating in Obese Rats, by PM Johnson and PJ Kenny, *Nature Neuroscience*, May 2010

9 Eating Soup Will Help Cut Calories at Meals, by B Rolls and J Flood, Penn State University, presented at the Experimental Biology Conference in Washington, May 2007

10 Vegetarian Diets and Weight Status, by SE Berkow and N Barnard, *Nutrition Reviews*, April 2006
Weight Gain over 5 Years in 21,966 Meat-eating, Fish-eating, Vegetarian, and Vegan Men and Women, by M Rosell, P Appleby, E Spencer and T Key, *International Journal of Obesity*, September 2006

11 Meat Consumption is Associated with Obesity and Central Obesity among US Adults, by Y Wang and MA Beydoun, *International Journal of Obesity*, June 2009

12 The Impact of Vitamin C Depletion on a Short-term Diet, by B Beezhold and C Johnston, Arizona State University, reported at Experimental Biology presentation in San Francisco, 2006

13 A Pavlovian Approach to the Problem of Obesity, by S Swithers and T Davidson, Purdue University, Indiana, *International Journal of Obesity*, June 2004

A Role for Sweet Taste: calorie predictive relations in energy regulation by rats, by SE Swithers and TL Davidson, Purdue University, *Behavioral Neuroscience*, February 2008

14 The Effect of Coffee on Blood Pressure and Cardiovascular Disease in Hypertensive Individuals, by AE Mesas, LM Leon-Munoz and E Lopez-Garcia, Department of Preventive Medicine and Public Health, Universidad Autónoma de Madrid, Spain, *American Journal of Clinical Nutrition*, 2011

Coffee Consumption and Risk of Stroke: a dose-response meta-analysis of prospective studies, by S Larsson and N Orsini, National Institute of Environmental Medicine, Karolinska Institutet, Stockholm, Sweden, *American Journal of Epidemiology*, September 2011

Coffee Consumption and Risk of Chronic Disease, by A Floegel, T Pischon, MM Bergmann, B Teucher, R Kaaks and H Boeing, European Prospective Investigation into Cancer and Nutrition, Germany, *American Journal of Clinical Nutrition*, 2012

15 Meta-analysis of Short Sleep Duration and Obesity in Children and Adults, by F Cappuccio, University of Warwick, *Sleep*, 2008

16 Short Sleep Duration is Associated with Reduced Leptin, Elevated Ghrelin, and Increased Body Mass Index, by S Taheri and E Mignot, Stanford University, Public Library of Science, *PLoS Medicine*, December 2004

17 The Mechanisms for the Interaction Between Sleep and Metabolism, by S Taheri, Bristol University, *International Journal of Sleep and Wakefulness*, 2007

18 Short Sleep Duration is Associated with Reduced Leptin Levels and Increased Adiposity: results from the Québec family study, by J-P Chaput, Laval University, Quebec, *Obesity*, January 2007

19 Super Bowls: Serving Bowl Size and Food Consumption, by B Wansink and MM. Cheney, *Journal of the American Medical Association*, April 2005

20 The Ecology of Eating: smaller portion sizes in France than in the United States help explain the French paradox, by P Rozin, *Psychological Science*, Sept 2003

21 The Perils of Plate Size: Waist, Waste, and Wallet, by B Wansink and K van Ittersum, *Journal of Marketing*, 2006

The Visual Illusions of Food: why plates, bowls, and spoons can bias consumption volume, *FASEB Journal*, 2006

22 Weight Loss During the Intensive Intervention Phase of the Weight-Loss Maintenance Trial, by JF Hollis et al, Kaiser Permanente's Center for Health Research, *American Journal of Preventive Medicine*, August 2008

23 Mindless Eating: the 200 daily food decisions we overlook, by B Wansink and J Sobal, *Environment and Behavior*, January 2007

24 The Office Candy Dish: proximity's influence on estimated and actual consumption, by B Wansink, JE Painter and Y-K Lee, *International Journal of Obesity*, May 2006

25 Bad Popcorn in Big Buckets: portion size can influence intake as much as taste, by B Wansink and J Kim, Cornell University, New York, *Journal of Nutrition Education and Behavior*, Sept/Oct 2005

Bottomless Bowls: why visual cues of portion size may influence intake, by B Wansink, JE Painter and J North, *Obesity Research*, 2005

26 The Effect of Distractions While Tasting a Food Sample, by B Shiv, *Journal of Consumer Research*, 2004

27 How Are Habits Formed: modelling habit formation in the real world, by P Lally, CHM van Jaarsveld, HWW Potts and J Wardlel, University College London, *European Journal of Social Psychology*, October2010

28 Automaticity in Situ: direct context cuing of habits in daily life, by W Wood, Duke University in North Carolina, quoted in the *New York Times*, 2007

29 How Positive And Negative Feedback Motivate Goal Pursuit, by A Fishbach, T Eyal and SR Finkelstein, *Social and Personality Psychology Compass*, 2010

30 From Passive Overeating to Food Addiction: a spectrum of compulsion and severity, by C Davis, York University, Toronto, Canada, *Obesity*, April 2013

31 Life Changes: How to Create New Habits, *Huffington Post*, November 2012, http://www.huffingtonpost.com/2012/11/26/life-changes-how-to-createhabits_n_1970105.html

32 Regulatory Accessibility and Social Influences on State Self-control, by MR Van Dellen and RH Hoyle, *Personality and Social Psychology Bulletin*, 2010

33 Beneficial Metabolic Adaptations Due to Endurance Exercise Training in the Fasted State, by K Van Proeyen et al, Research Centre for Exercise and Health, Department of Biomedical Kinesiology, Leuven, Belgium, *Journal of Applied Physiology*, January 2011

34 Acute Effects of a Single Exercise Class on Appetite, Energy Intake and Mood. Is there a time of day effect? By M Maraki et al, University of Glasgow, *Appetite*, December 2005

35 Training in the Fasted State Improves Glucose Tolerance during Fat-Rich Diet, by K Van Proeyen et al, Research Centre for Exercise and Health, Department of Biomedical Kinesiology, Leuven, Belgium, *Journal of Physiology*, November 2010

36 Adaptations to Skeletal Muscle with Endurance Exercise Training in the

Acutely Fed Versus Overnight-Fasted State, by SR Stannard, AJ Buckley, JA Edge and MW Thompson, *Journal of Science and Medicine in Sport*, July 2010

37 The Effect of High-Intensity Intermittent Exercise on Body Composition of Overweight Young Males, M Heydari, J Freund and SH Boutcher, *Journal of Obesity*, June 2012

38 Physiological Adaptations to Low-Volume, High-Intensity Interval Training in Health and Disease, by MJ Gibala, JP Little, MJ Macdonald and JA Hawley, *Journal of Physiology*, January 2012

39 Metabolic and Behavioral Compensatory Responses to Exercise Interventions: barriers to weight loss, by NA King et al, *Obesity*, June 2007

40 'Just Thinking about Exercise Makes Me Serve More Food': physical activity and calorie compensation, by CC Werle, B Wansink and CR Payne, Cornell University, *Appetite*, September 2011

41 Towards the Minimal Amount of Exercise for Improving Metabolic Health, by RS Metcalfe, JA Babraj, SG Fawkner, and NB Vollaard, *European Journal of Applied Physiology*, July 2012

42 Low-Volume Interval Training Improves Muscle Oxidative Capacity in Sedentary Adults, by MS Hood et al, *Medicine & Science in Sports & Exercise*, October 2011

43 The 24-hour Energy Intake of Obese Adolescents is Spontaneously Reduced after Intensive Exercise: a randomized controlled trial in calorimetric chambers, by P Duché and B Morio, *International Journal of Obesity*, June 2013

44 Will Alsop quote from the *Guardian*, January 2007

45 The Geneva Stair Study, by P Meyer, University Hospital of Geneva, September 2008

46 Sanex Walk for Skin 2008, study of sitting, reported in the *Daily Mail*, April 2008

47 Role of Low Energy Expenditure and Sitting in Obesity, Metabolic Syndrome, Type 2 Diabetes, and Cardiovascular Disease, by MT Hamilton, University of Missouri-Columbia, *Diabetes*, September 2007

48 Obesity Relationships with Community Design, Physical Activity and Time Spent in Cars, by L Frank, University of British Columbia, *American Journal of Preventive Medicine*, June 2002

49 Using Pedometers to Increase Physical Activity and Improve Health: a systematic review, by DM Bravata, Stanford University, *Journal of the American Medical Association*, November 2007

50 Mind-Set Matters: exercise and the placebo effect, by A Crum and E Langer, Department of Psychology, Harvard University, *Psychological Science*, February 2007

index

ACKNOWLEDGEMENTS

My thanks, as always, go to Dr Michael Mosley, originator of the 5:2 Diet and a constantly inspiring companion on this remarkable adventure. Thank you, too, to my friends Rebecca Nicolson and Aurea Carpenter, and to the ever-fantastic Fast Diet team – Paul Bougourd, Emmie Francis, Klara Zak, Catherine Gibbs, Georgia Vaux, Dr Sarah Schenker and Annie Hudson. I'd also like to offer my personal thanks to the many people who have shared their 5:2 stories with us. In the last instance, it is your progress towards health and well-being that underpins all that we do. Closer to home, my family deserves a huge hug for putting up with a mother who is sometimes (but not always) too busy to bake cakes.

---

www.thefastdiet.co.uk
@mimispencer1
@thefastdietbook
www.facebook.co.uk/thefastdiet.co.uk
And look out for the Fast Beach Diet app

Mimi Spencer has written about body shape, diet and food trends in national newspapers and magazines for more than 20 years. She co-authored **The Fast Diet** (Short Books, 2013) with Dr Michael Mosley, and wrote **The Fast Diet Recipe Book** (Short Books, 2013) and **Fast Cook** (2014).

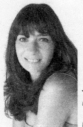

Dave Poole